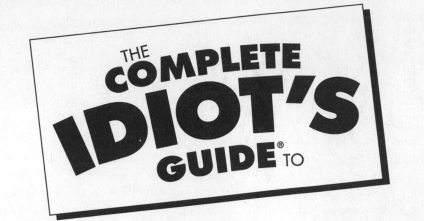

THE COMPLETE IDIOT'S GUIDE TO

Lowering Your Cholesterol

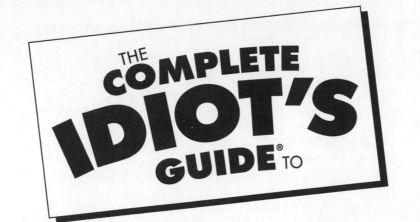

THE
COMPLETE IDIOT'S GUIDE® TO

Lowering Your Cholesterol

by Joseph Lee Klapper, M.D.

A member of Penguin Group (USA) Inc.

To Regina, Elijah, Jeremiah, Sarah, Mom and Dad, and Alan and Alicia

ALPHA BOOKS

Published by the Penguin Group

Penguin Group (USA) Inc., 375 Hudson Street, New York, New York 10014, U.S.A.

Penguin Group (Canada), 10 Alcorn Avenue, Toronto, Ontario, Canada M4V 3B2 (a division of Pearson Penguin Canada Inc.)

Penguin Books Ltd, 80 Strand, London WC2R 0RL, England

Penguin Ireland, 25 St Stephen's Green, Dublin 2, Ireland (a division of Penguin Books Ltd)

Penguin Group (Australia), 250 Camberwell Road, Camberwell, Victoria 3124, Australia (a division of Pearson Australia Group Pty Ltd)

Penguin Books India Pvt Ltd, 11 Community Centre, Panchsheel Park, New Delhi—110 017, India

Penguin Group (NZ), cnr Airborne and Rosedale Roads, Albany, Auckland 1310, New Zealand (a division of Pearson New Zealand Ltd)

Penguin Books (South Africa) (Pty) Ltd, 24 Sturdee Avenue, Rosebank, Johannesburg 2196, South Africa

Penguin Books Ltd, Registered Offices: 80 Strand, London WC2R 0RL, England

Publisher: *Marie Butler-Knight*
Editorial Director: *Mike Sanders*
Managing Editor: *Billy Fields*
Executive Editor: *Randy Ladenheim-Gil*
Development Editor: *Ginny Bess Munroe*
Senior Production Editor: *Janette Lynn*
Copy Editor: *Michael Dietsch*

Cartoonist: *Shannon Wheeler*
Cover Designer: *Bill Thomas*
Book Designers: *Trina Wurst/Kurt Owens*
Indexer: *Julie Bess*
Layout: *Brian Massey*
Proofreader: *Mary Hunt*

Contents at a Glance

Contents

Introduction

Americans are more aware of health and healthy living than ever before, so why is it that cholesterol levels continue to rise and unhealthy habits (such as smoking, eating fast food and leading a sedentary lifestyle) persist? All these factors can cause elevated cholesterol levels, which, as you'll read in this book, can in turn lead to serious health consequences.

The purpose of this book is to help you achieve better health; the first step in that quest is to adapt a healthy lifestyle. Regular exercise combined with a low-fat diet can help to reduce cholesterol level and reduce your risk of illness. The best part of learning how to lower your risk for cardiovascular disease is that you'll also be improving your overall health: the measures I advise for lowering your risk of illness will also help you to lose weight and increase your energy level!

Improving your health is not an impossible venture. No matter how many times you've tried and not succeeded at changing your lifestyle, it's never too late to try again. Think of those previous attempts as proof that you *can* do it; you just need to take it to the next level this time! *Permanent* lifestyle changes, including a low-fat diet and regular exercise, are the goal; the tools you'll need for reaching those goals don't include an expensive home gym or a personal chef. All you need is the desire to correct (or mitigate) the damage that cholesterol has already done inside your arteries. If you have that, you'll find that it's relatively easy to take the necessary steps toward a healthier you!

How to Use This Book

In order to help you appreciate the damage that occurs in the presence of elevated cholesterol levels, this book starts out by discussing the different kinds of cholesterol and what they do to the arteries and the body. We'll then move on to specific tips and advice for improving health.

Part 1, The Heart of the Problem, takes a look at each type of cholesterol. Not all cholesterol is created equally; unfortunately, most people with elevated cholesterol tend to have high amounts of the "bad" type, which can cause all sorts of misery inside the arteries and, by extension, throughout the body. This section also includes a breakdown of risk factors that increase a person's risk for developing cardiovascular disease and tests that are commonly used for diagnostic purposes.

Part 2, Nutrition for Lowering Cholesterol, gives you all kinds of ideas (and reasons) for tossing out your high-fat foods and replacing them with lighter, healthier fare! A major part of this section centers on eating foods in their most natural forms.

I'll tell you which kinds of food may help to lower cholesterol levels, where to find them, and how to ensure that you're using them properly for the best possible health results.

Part 3, Mind and Body Approaches for Lowering Cholesterol, provides strategies for reducing stress and improving physical fitness. One important fact about heart health: the "good" cholesterol, HDL, may increase in response to physical activity; furthermore, levels of the "bad" cholesterol, LDL, can be lowered by regular exercise! You'll read about easy ways to work meditation and activity into your regular daily routine.

Part 4, Medications and Natural Remedies, gets into the slightly more complex issues of medicinal help for lowering cholesterol. In this section, you'll read about medications that are commonly used for the purpose of decreasing cholesterol levels. And because herbs and nutritional supplements are very popular these days, I'll also discuss the merits of using some of these natural compounds.

Part 5, Dr. Klapper's Step-by-Step Guide to Losing Cholesterol Points, includes specific advice that I give to my own patients, including why I prefer specific medications, what I have to say on the topic of smoking, and at what age a person should ideally have his or her first cholesterol screening.

I've also included three appendixes: the first is a glossary. Even though I've broken this book down into the simplest terms, this is a medical topic. Since I don't want you to get lost in the language or confused by any of the terms, the definitions are all compiled for easy reference in Appendix A. Flip back to them whenever you need to. Appendix B includes articles and books that I have used in my own research and that you may find helpful in your quest to learn more about cholesterol. And in Appendix C, you'll find a selection of easy-to-prepare recipes—main and side dishes, and desserts and snacks—that will get you cooking with such flavor boosters as herbs and spices, as well as low-fat ingredients like vinegar and mustard.

Extras

Improving your health might seem like a complicated issue, so to simplify things as much as possible, this book uses four different kinds of margin notes to pull out important information and bring it to your immediate attention:

Healthy Heart Facts
Stories, studies, and facts related to cardiovascular health.

Here's to Your Heart

Food, exercise, and lifestyle tips aimed at improving your heart's health.

def•i•ni•tion

Definitions of cholesterol-related terms and phrases used in the adjacent text.

The Doctor Says

Warnings and cautions about potentially dangerous conditions and situations.

Acknowledgments

The following people were instrumental in helping to nurture and develop this project: Jacky Sach, my agent at Bookends Literary Agency; Randy Ladenheim-Gil, executive editor, and Ginny Munroe, development editor, and Mike Dietsch, copy editor, at Alpha Books. A (healthy) heartfelt thanks to each of you! A warm thanks also goes to Meghan Beecher for supplying some of the delicious and healthy recipes in Appendix C.

Trademarks

Part 1

The Heart of the Problem

It seems as though everyone you know is trying to lower their cholesterol levels—and maybe your doctor has suggested that you follow suit. But why? What is it about cholesterol that makes it such a hazard to your health?

Most people are mainly concerned with how "bad" cholesterol might affect their health. In the following chapters, we break cholesterol down into its most basic components, discuss how to raise "good" cholesterol and lower the "bad" stuff, talk about risk factors associated with heart disease and stroke, and learn about how cholesterol abnormalities are diagnosed. You'll come away from this reading feeling as though you've learned more information about cholesterol than you knew existed, which is a good thing. This isn't tough stuff to understand … but understanding it could mean the difference between having good health and serious health problems!

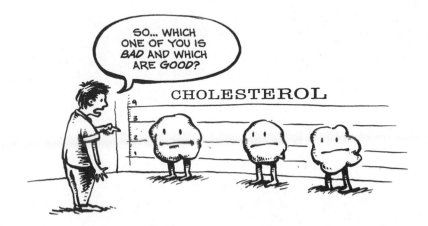

Understanding Cholesterol

In This Chapter

◆ Discover the components and functions of cholesterol

◆ Learn why we need cholesterol

◆ Understand cholesterol's effects on blood vessels

◆ Familiarize yourself with healthy cholesterol levels

When we use the word *cholesterol*, what are we really talking about? Some mysterious measurement of the blood? Some random number scale that doctors created to cause the common man undue angst? You might say, "I'm lowering my cholesterol," or, "My cholesterol levels are sky-high," but how often do you stop and define cholesterol for yourself?

When we talk about cholesterol, we're essentially talking about fat in the bloodstream. You might be thinking, "That's strange. Fat doesn't belong in the bloodstream." *Now* you're getting the picture! This chapter talks about what is cholesterol, why we actually need some of it, and how and why it can cause major heartache—literally.

What Is Cholesterol?

Cholesterol is a steroid-like substance derived from the food you eat and modified by the liver. Basically, it's a fatty substance that will not dissolve in the bloodstream. Cholesterol plays an important role in maintaining certain bodily functions, which we discuss later in this chapter. What you need to know for now is that cholesterol needs to reach certain organs, so that they perform their functions.

The way cholesterol works in the body is interesting, although fairly complex, so it's broken down into several steps for easier understanding.

♦ Cholesterol is absorbed in the intestine and travels through special blood vessels that take it directly to the liver, which packages the cholesterol by coating it with a protein envelope. These protein coats determine to which organs the cholesterol packages will travel.

♦ As the cholesterol packages attach themselves to various tissues and organs by their protein coats, they deposit some of their cholesterol cores into the tissues and organs. After the particles have deposited their cholesterol and other fatty substances that are contained in their cores, they become new packages. These new packages then travel back to the liver and are modified further.

♦ Cholesterol that the organs and tissues do not use is eventually released into the stool through the bile. The liver produces bile, which contains various enzymes needed for digestion as well as waste products for disposal, such as cholesterol.

So you see, there's more to cholesterol than the bad name it gets in medical reports. Cholesterol travels between various tissues and the liver, shuttling back and forth, depositing cholesterol within various body parts where it is needed. You could say that cholesterol is a busy and vital part of the body's day-to-day operations!

def•i•ni•tion

Cholesterol is a fatty substance that does not dissolve in the bloodstream. Although cholesterol is needed for some of the body's basic functions, it can also pose serious health risks if it damages the blood vessels.

A **cholesterol panel** measures the amount of fatty substances, or lipids, in the blood. The substances measured in a cholesterol panel include HDL, LDL, and triglycerides, and are sometimes referred to as **subfractions** or **lipid subfractions**. Measurements are reported in mg/dl, which is a reflection of the concentration of cholesterol in the bloodstream.

Break It Down

When your cholesterol is measured in your doctor's office, that test is called a *cholesterol panel.* You don't just get one number back on this test; cholesterol is broken down into various *subfractions* that indicate how well—or how poorly—your arteries may be holding up. The three major subfractions that doctors are concerned with are LDL (low-density lipoproteins), HDL (high-density lipoproteins), and triglycerides.

> **Healthy Heart Facts**
>
> LDL is called the *bad* cholesterol, and HDL is the *good* cholesterol. Triglycerides are lipids that may be contained in the core of cholesterol. We talk more about these individual substances in Chapters 2, 3, and 4, respectively.

So what makes one cholesterol "good" and another one "bad"? It all comes down to their specific protein coating, as well as their cholesterol contents. LDL, for example, is coated by a protein containing a substance called APO B-100. This substance is recognized by receptors on various cells, tissues, and organs; LDL goes looking for these receptors. After it finds them, it binds itself to them, allowing cholesterol to accumulate inside blood vessels. This accumulation of blood vessels increases the future risk of heart attack and stroke.

While bad cholesterol can do horrendous things to the arteries, the body also needs cholesterol in order to survive. That's right—this cholesterol, which you hear such terrible reports about, is actually *needed* (to some degree) by your internal organs. We talk about bad cholesterol in more detail later in this chapter.

> **Healthy Heart Facts**
>
> Ever wonder who decides how high or low cholesterol target numbers should be? The Adult Treatment Panel of the National Cholesterol Program (NCEP/ATP) of the National Heart, Lung and Blood Institute (Whew! Out of breath just reading that? Try typing it!) makes these calls. This is a public recommendation updated periodically. Even though the latest recommendations were updated recently (in 2004), things change so quickly in medicine that we need another full update to these guidelines already!

Spin Zone

You can tell more about blood and its components—including cholesterol—by performing various lab tests. In one such test, the cholesterol in the bloodstream is separated from the blood in the form of a creamy, fatty substance. The blood is spun down, or centrifuged, separating the cholesterol from the blood. The cholesterol will settle according to its density. So, for example, the low-density cholesterol, or LDL (the bad cholesterol), is more buoyant than the high-density cholesterol, or HDL (the good cholesterol).

The buoyant cholesterol separates to the top of the creamy supernatant (which is the fluid that's left after that spinning finishes), while the denser components end up at the bottom. The centrifuge machine separates the cholesterol components from blood based upon its heaviness or density in water.

Healthy Heart Facts

LDL cholesterol is more dangerous than HDL cholesterol, which is generally protective and reduces the risk of heart attack and stroke. Typically, there is far more LDL traveling in the bloodstream than necessary, which deposits excess cholesterol inside of the blood vessels. HDL, meanwhile, can act as a vacuum to clean out the LDL, but only if HDL levels are higher than LDL levels. We discuss these cholesterol subfractions in more detail in Chapters 2 and 3.

Why You Need Cholesterol

With all the talk about lowering cholesterol and the scary health risks associated with out-of-control cholesterol levels, you might be thinking, "Hey, let's just get rid of it all together! I mean, who *needs* it?" Well, you do. And I do. Everyone needs a certain amount of cholesterol in order to survive. And what's more, because cholesterol plays a role in hormone production, we can also say that the propagation of the human species depends on cholesterol! Because cholesterol is the starting point for sex steroid hormone synthesis, without cholesterol, sex hormone production and reproduction would not be possible. Let's break this down to a basic level: every cell in the body is surrounded by a cell membrane. Cells communicate with each other and their environment using these membranes. Guess what substance is a basic component of cell membranes? You know it—cholesterol. So, without exaggeration, we can say that without cholesterol, our lives wouldn't be possible. Now, some people feel that it's impossible to live life without *added* cholesterol—in the form of burgers, fries, and milkshakes—but that's another argument all together, and one that this book dismantles. The following illustration gives you an idea of how cells "talk" to each other, and why cell membrane health is so important to our very existence!

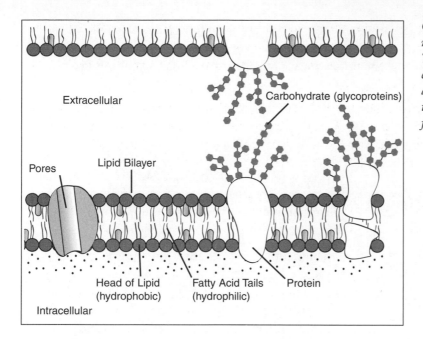

Cholesterol is needed for cell membrane development. These membranes allow for cells to interact with one another in order to perform the most basic life-sustaining functions.

Because cholesterol is needed to sustain cell life at its most rudimentary level, it also plays a role to sustain our major bodily functions and organs, such as the brain, heart, and nerves. It also plays a role in the production of steroid hormones, such as testosterone, estrogen, and progesterone, each of which is important in reproduction.

Healthy Heart Facts

Years ago, autopsies of Vietnam and Korean War casualties (generally young, healthy males) noted fatty, cholesterol laden deposits within certain areas of the blood vessels. Upon further examination, the aorta (the main artery that delivers blood from the heart to the rest of the body) was almost always found to contain deposits of fat within its walls, called fatty streaks. These streaks are the earliest manifestations of cholesterol deposits. Now, this type of cardiovascular damage was not limited to Korean War casualties; fatty streaks have been observed in young people of every generation. The thing to remember about these studies is this: cholesterol starts doing its damage at an early age, in people who appear to be completely healthy!

Symptoms of High Cholesterol

The first symptoms of elevated cholesterol aren't really symptoms at all, but rather what we could call findings. For example, when cholesterol begins to deposit itself on the inner lining of the blood vessels, it doesn't cause any symptoms per se. It's only when the damage has been done (for example, these deposits encourage the formation of a blood clot that later breaks loose and causes a heart attack or stroke) that symptoms occur.

Inflammatory Evidence

When we talk about elevated cholesterol levels, we need to talk about *inflammation*, which is the body's response to an infection or a foreign body. When inflammation occurs, cells called *macrophages* rush to the site of an infection to stop bacteria dead in its tracks. Macrophages help defend the body from uncontrolled infection by actually eating the bacteria.

def•i•ni•tion

> **Inflammation** is the body's response to an infection. Specialized cells called **macrophages** are sent out to control the bacteria and shut down the infection. Cholesterol can also act as an inflammatory substance and cause inflammation.

Inflammation has a negative connotation, probably because when a person has an inflammation, he or she may be ill and likely in pain from the swelling that often accompanies this macrophage picnic. But in reality, inflammation is something that helps you survive. It's the body's way of fighting off infection, and it's actually going on inside the body all the time to some degree. Without inflammation, you would succumb to nasty bacteria and die. Think of inflammation as a slow burn. It's only when that slow burn gets out of control and spreads that you should think of inflammation as a destructive wildfire.

So how does this relate to cholesterol? Inflammation is usually a response to bacterial invasion; however, cholesterol can also act as an inflammatory substance and initiate a macrophage attack. The macrophages die after eating up the cholesterol and then release an enzyme that damages the inner lining of the blood vessels. As a result, the blood vessels cannot supply blood to the organs as well as they should. The skin, brain, heart, and muscles are all affected by this poor perfusion of blood.

Clotting

Clotting is actually a component of inflammation, and like inflammation, is one of those bodily functions that's necessary for survival, but it can also cause major health problems if it spirals out of control.

Think about what happens when you cut your finger. The blood flows for a moment and then stops. Your clotting system has rushed to the scene of the injury and helped to stem the flow of blood. Ideally, clots are localized—they only show up when and where they're needed, just like inflammation. And when the clotting system springs into action, an anticlotting system also goes to work to prevent the clot from spreading.

When there's either too much clotting or too much anticlotting, people can run into health problems. And unfortunately, cholesterol can contribute to an overabundance of clotting. Let's talk about what happens when someone has a heart attack. The cholesterol that has already damaged the lining of the blood vessel is lying underneath that lining in a liquid pool that also contains dead macrophages and other by-products of inflammation. The pool is prevented from entering into the bloodstream by a cap that is sitting on top of it. The combination of the liquid pool and the cap is called *plaque*; this plaque forms throughout the body in people who have elevated cholesterol levels.

The Doctor Says

Human bodies are really in a continuous state of clotting, as small blood clots are always forming near cholesterol-rich areas of our blood vessels. Thankfully, the anticlotting system is able to dismantle these tiny clots and prevent them from becoming massive enough to cause heart attacks and strokes.

def•i•ni•tion

Plaque forms on blood vessel walls. It's made up of a liquid pool containing cholesterol and by-products of inflammation as well as a protective cap that prevents the cholesterol from entering into the bloodstream.

The cholesterol in this pool, meanwhile, is highly inflammatory and also highly effective at triggering a massive blood clot. When there is some stressor on the plaque surface, the plaque, being soft and fragile, ruptures and releases its central contents—the cholesterol pool—into the bloodstream. This cholesterol pool is highly inflammatory to flowing blood and extremely effective at causing the blood to clot.

This clot grows like a snowball rolling down a mountainside, eventually forming an avalanche of clotting. When this massive clot fills the inside of an artery supplying heart muscle, a heart attack occurs. A stroke occurs when this clot occludes an artery supplying blood to the brain.

Any disruption in the protective cap can allow the cholesterol to enter the bloodstream and trigger a clot, which, in turn, can cause a heart attack or stroke.

Cholesterol Makes You Old

The aging process is predetermined by a complex genetic code, which tells us that the human body is designed to break down and die in an orderly fashion. Even if people lead healthy lifestyles, cells eventually start to fall apart and they will develop diseases, such as cancer or heart disease. This is why people can't live forever—the body just won't allow it. But this is also why you usually see certain conditions (such as heart disease) in elderly people. It's just nature's way of shutting down the body.

Every single cell plays a part in the aging process. And because every cell depends on blood circulation for its own optimum health, we know that healthy blood vessels are necessary for a healthy body. Our overall health is determined by the health of the inner lining of every blood vessel in our bodies.

When your blood vessels aren't performing well, your organs don't receive an adequate amount of blood, and the aging process actually speeds up, which leads to poor health. On the other hand, reducing cholesterol levels helps to salvage the blood vessels, and this maintains youth to some degree.

So you don't really need Botox or a makeover to feel younger—you can start by lowering your cholesterol!

Causes of High Cholesterol

There are really two causes of elevated cholesterol levels: genetics and environment. This means that although your family may have passed down a less-than-healthy cholesterol history, your lifestyle can be an equal contributor to your high LDL levels.

Most Americans with high cholesterol can attribute their problem to a typical Western diet superimposed on a family history. So before you blame your mom and dad for your health problems, ask yourself if you've really been leading the healthiest lifestyle. Chances are you could be doing better.

Heart Attack on a Plate with a Side of Fries

The primary cause of elevated cholesterol levels is a diet high in saturated fats. Because we in the Western world love fried foods and red meats, it's really no wonder that we also seem to love our elevated cholesterol levels.

All right, maybe *loving* elevated LDL is a bit of a stretch, but you'd never know it based on the typical Western diet, which includes enough fat to … well, to clog an artery or two!

Foods that contribute to elevated cholesterol levels include …

◆ **Fatty meats**—Like your bacon? Your arteries don't. Sausage, fried chicken, marbled beef—they're all full of fat and bad for your health!

◆ **Fried foods**—French fries, fried chicken, fried fish … so good and yet so bad for you.

◆ **Baked foods**—Pastries, in particular, are loaded with fat and cholesterol.

◆ **Dairy products**—Whole milk, heavy cream, ice cream, and cheese all contribute to elevated cholesterol. Look for their low-fat or skim counterparts.

◆ **Processed foods**—You're not helping your heart by using nondairy creamer. It's loaded with additives that are terrible for your arteries. Any food that uses a lot of preserving agents is, as a rule of thumb, not very good for you.

Don't complicate matters by making a list of foods that you shouldn't eat. Essentially, it's easier to consider what's good for you rather than focusing on what's bad. Lean meats (such as fish, poultry, and occasionally, lean beef) are doctor-approved. And you can't go wrong with fruits and vegetables; it's not really possible to overeat fruits and vegetables. The more of these you work into your diet, the better.

Don't Blame Your Parents!

Certain genetic defects can leave someone predisposed to serious cholesterol problems. For example, a certain genetic defect of the liver makes it impossible for the body to clear LDL from the bloodstream. This condition can lead to LDL levels of over 500 (sometimes in the thousands!), and can lead to heart attacks even in young patients.

It's difficult to assign high cholesterol as a genetic problem, though, because doctors can never really be sure how much of a person's family history is due to genetics and how much is due to lifestyle choices. In other words, it may seem obvious to you that you have been dealt a bad genetic hand when it comes to heart disease and high cholesterol: your parents both died of heart attacks, and so did your maternal grandfather and your paternal grandmother. But…did they consume fried foods a little too often? Were they each devoted to consuming a half-gallon of ice cream nightly? Did any of them dedicate themselves to an exercise routine?

You can see how tough it is to determine where genetics leave off and environment takes over. We do know, however, that in the last century, average cholesterol levels have gone up in the United States, and this is most likely because of environmental factors, which really refers to diet.

Cholesterol Levels and Your Health

The effects of cholesterol on health depend on how many other risk factors a person has for developing illness. Risk factors for heart attack and stroke are covered in detail in Chapter 5. They include …

- ◆ Genetics.
- ◆ Age.
- ◆ Gender.
- ◆ Diet.
- ◆ Exercise.

Adding up a person's risk factors produces a *baseline risk*. When high cholesterol is superimposed on an elevated baseline risk, then the adverse effects of high cholesterol become magnified.

def•i•ni•tion

A person's **baseline risk** for heart attack and stroke is determined by evaluating their risk for developing these conditions, such as diet, exercise, gender, age, and genetics. If a baseline risk is already high, an elevated cholesterol level can make matters even worse.

Let's use an extreme example to illustrate baseline risk and cholesterol: two people have a total cholesterol level of 200 (with an LDL level of 160). The first person is a 60-year-old male who consumes a high-fat diet and who has diabetes, obesity, and high blood pressure. The second person is a 21-year-old female marathon runner who consumes a vegan diet and who is of normal weight. The 60-year-old male is at much higher risk for developing a heart attack or stroke because he has so many *other* risk factors.

Multiple Risks

Interestingly, many risk factors for heart disease tend to track together in individuals. In other words, a person who has high cholesterol often has other health problems that can contribute to the development of heart disease.

Some of these risk factors include …

- ◆ Obesity or being overweight.
- ◆ Diabetes.
- ◆ Sedentary lifestyle.

♦ High-fat diet.

♦ High blood pressure.

Frequently, though, heart attacks happen to people who have only mildly elevated cholesterol and no other risk factors. Because risk factors seem to play such a big role in heart disease, how could this happen? Well, for one thing, in the United States and Western Europe, what we deem acceptable cholesterol levels are well above where cholesterol levels should ideally be. In fact, as researchers learn more about cholesterol, the target numbers for acceptable cholesterol levels continue to drop. The following chart gives you an idea of where the current guidelines lie and reflects LDL cholesterol goals and cut-off points for the initiation of cholesterol-lowering medication and diet.

Risk Category	LDL Goal (mg LDL)	LDL Level at which to Initiate Therapeutic Lifestyle Change (TLC) (mg LDL)	LDL Level at which to Consider Drug Therapy (mg LDL)
CHD or CHD Risk Equivalents (10 yr. Risk >20%)	<100	≥100	≥130 (100–129: Drug Optional)
2 + Risk Factors (10 yr. Risk ≤ 20%)	<130	≥130	10 yr. Risk 10–20%: ≥130 10 yr. Risk 10% ≥160
0 – 1 Risk Factor	<160	≥160	≥100 (160 – 189: LDL-lowering Drug Optional)

These 10-year Risk Categories are derived from the Framingham Study.
Risk Categories: ≤10% Low Risk, 10–20% Intermediate Risk, ≥20% High Risk.

It's also possible for someone to have a risk factor (or two) that they aren't even aware of. High blood pressure, for example, is silent, painless, and potentially deadly. In fact, these hidden risk factors often aren't discovered *until* someone has a heart attack or stroke. For this reason, it's important that elevated cholesterol be treated aggressively all the time.

Risk? What Risk?

Patients who have a normal cholesterol reading (HDL and LDL levels totaling under 200) are often lulled into a sense of complacency, figuring they're at low risk and can afford to eat high-fat foods, ignore their exercise routine, or even stop taking their cholesterol-lowering medications. However, doctors are learning more about cholesterol than ever before, and that includes how cholesterol is broken down. We know, for example, that HDL levels should be nice and high and LDL levels should be as low as possible.

Let's say a patient with a known cholesterol level of 190 comes into the emergency room suffering from a heart attack. The doctors will measure his cholesterol level during the heart attack, and it might come back at 180 (which is normal; cholesterol can drop during a heart attack). Upon further investigation, however, they may find that although this man's LDL level is 90 (acceptable level—it's below 100, which is ideal), his HDL level is only 18! *This* is what placed him at high risk for developing a heart attack in the first place! (Remember, HDL is the good, protective cholesterol.) We'll discuss LDL and HDL in more detail in Chapters 2 and 3, respectively.

The Doctor Says

Doctors are learning that LDL, or the bad cholesterol, can be broken down into components, and that each component carries a different level of risk. For example, one type of LDL, called *small dense LDL,* can raise one's risk of heart attack or stroke. The problem here is that a person can have a low LDL level, which we normally think is good; however, if the LDL are of the *small dense* type, that person has an elevated risk for heart attack and stroke.

The Good News

Yes, there is some good news! Cholesterol *can* be lowered. And simply put, the lower your cholesterol, the healthier you're likely to be—and remain.

Although lowering your cholesterol takes diligence (in the form of permanent changes to your lifestyle), the methods of cholesterol reduction (adopting a healthier diet, engaging in an exercise routine, quitting smoking) are relatively risk-free. And in the end, along with lower cholesterol, you'll achieve good health and longevity!

The Least You Need to Know

- ◆ Cholesterol refers to the steroid-like fatty substance present in the bloodstream.

- ◆ Cholesterol is divided into lipid subfractions, including LDL, HDL, and tri-glycerides.

- ◆ The human body needs some cholesterol to perform its basic functions.

- ◆ The number one cause of elevated cholesterol is a high-fat diet.

- ◆ Inflammation can result from having too much cholesterol in the bloodstream; this inflammation can lead to clotting, which, in turn can lead to heart attack and stroke.

LDL: The Bad Cholesterol

In This Chapter

- ◆ Read how LDL is formed
- ◆ Discover the harmful effects of LDL on your health
- ◆ Find out how low your LDL level should be
- ◆ Learn about fat and LDL
- ◆ See which foods are easily transformed into LDL

Chapter 1 mentioned that there are two types of cholesterol—the good kind and the bad kind. LDL is, as the title of this chapter suggests, the harmful type of cholesterol.

The primary focus of cholesterol reduction should be reducing LDL levels as much as possible. Studies have shown that reducing LDL levels reduces the risk of death because of heart attack and stroke, whether one has multiple risk factors or not. In reality, we all probably have a risk factor or two that we don't even know about, so even if you're feeling fine, lowering your LDL will work to your benefit. (And at any rate, it's certainly not going to do you any harm!)

What Is LDL?

LDL, or *low-density lipoprotein,* is one component of the cholesterol and fats circulating in the blood. LDL is a spherical complex combination of protein and cholesterol.

def•i•ni•tion

LDL stands for **low-density lipo-protein.** The role of LDL is to move cholesterol and other fatty compounds that are in excess to places where it can be stored.

All the fatty compounds derived from our food and made from our liver circulate in the bloodstream as particles. If you can picture how oil and water don't mix, it's easy to envision how cholesterol needs some sort special covering to help it blend in with the bloodstream. As oil floats to the surface of water, cholesterol (and similar fatty compounds) would also float to the surface of blood if it weren't for a mechanism to enhance its solubilization.

After fat is absorbed into the intestine, it makes its way to the liver. Some of the fat is removed there; the leftover fat travels in the blood in the form of *chylomicrons.* The liver manufactures LDL from the chylomicron remnants. LDL consists of cholesterol surrounded by a protein coat, which allows it to move through the bloodstream.

LDL is recognized by specific receptors on cells that need cholesterol. When cells require more cholesterol for basic functions, they express more receptors, or docking sites, on their surface to bind more LDL. As a result, LDL levels in the blood decrease. In a compensatory fashion, the liver may make more LDL. However, when the LDL supply circulating the blood is greater than the basic needs of the cells, the excess cholesterol is deposited within the inside of blood vessels as plaque.

Healthy Heart Facts

One way cholesterol-reducing medication works is by increasing the number of LDL receptors in the liver. This allows the liver to take in more of the cholesterol circulating as LDL in the bloodstream. As a result, less LDL is available to deposit in the arteries as plaque.

The body has difficulty ridding itself of excess cholesterol. Only a certain amount of excess cholesterol can be moved from the liver to the intestines and out through the stool each day. Excess cholesterol and other fatty compounds circulate in the blood as LDL and end up being deposited on the inside of blood vessels, which isn't the best place to dump these waste products.

LDL and Lowering Cholesterol

The goal of cholesterol reduction is to drop LDL levels as low as possible. Let's talk about a typical case. Someone with an LDL level of 190 *mg/dl* and no other risk factors for heart disease and stroke (such as obesity, diabetes, or high blood pressure) may be advised to lower his LDL to 160 mg/dl. If this same person had several risk factors, he would be advised to lower his LDL levels to 130 mg/dl.

Someone who already has heart disease (a person has already had a heart attack, for example), had a stroke, or has diabetes might be advised to drop his LDL to 100 mg/dl—but this recommendation would be based on somewhat outdated information. Personally, I would advise this person to shoot for an LDL level of 70 mg/dl or less, following the guidelines for very high risk patients set forth by the NCEP/ATP III (which publishes guidelines for cholesterol target numbers) in 2001 and updated in 2004.

As you can see, LDL is hardly held in high esteem—doctors want to see it go lower, lower, lower! In fact, from the current research, we may just find that there is no lower target number for LDL.

def•i•ni•tion

Cholesterol levels are measured by **mg/dl**, or *milligrams per deciliter*. You don't have to go back to high school and brush up on your metric system in order to understand these terms! Mg/dl is a simply measurement of the concentration of cholesterol in the blood. The higher the number (say, 200 mg/dl versus 130 mg/dl), the greater the threat to your health.

The Lowdown on LDL

Newborns have an LDL level between 25 and 40 mg/dl; meanwhile, the average American adult's LDL level is somewhere between 130 and 160 mg/dl.

Studies are showing us that there's no reason that LDL needs to increase with age; it doesn't do us any good. In fact, the opposite is true—LDL is harmful to the body and increases the risk of serious illness. It's likely that one day, doctors will find that these newborn LDL levels are ideal for adults, as well, and even lower levels of LDL will be the recommended norm.

Here's to Your Heart

Studies have shown that a reduction in LDL leads to a linear reduction in mortality (death rates). What does that mean, in lay terms? Your chances of leading a long and healthy life can be increased if you decrease your LDL. This point isn't even disputable; it's a basic, unchallenged fact in medicine.

What LDL Does to the Arteries

LDL floats around in the bloodstream until it's recognized by cells on the inner lining of the arteries. These arteries are important in the grand scheme of things, because they lead to the heart, kidneys, legs, eyes, and abdominal organs (stomach, liver, intestines).

Arteries have receptors inside of them that are made from sugar and protein. In fact, these receptors cover the surface of the inner lining of the blood vessels, or the endothelial cells, which are in constant contact with flowing blood. LDL attaches itself to the lining of these blood vessels and encourages the formation of plaque, which causes the damage.

All of us can—and do—live with some degree of plaque buildup on the inside of our arteries. People who have elevated cholesterol levels, however, have more plaque development than people who have normal cholesterol levels. Even substantial amounts of plaque can cause few or possibly no symptoms, however, because the arteries are able to make certain adaptations for survival.

For example, an artery can be up to 40 percent narrowed by plaque and appear normal on an angiogram. This is because the artery enlarges, or compensates, for the problem. Plus, blockages that develop over many years allow the heart to form collaterals, or auto-bypasses, around the blockages (we'll talk more about this in the following section). Because of this, people with high cholesterol levels can remain symptom free for many years. Of course, just because someone is symptom free doesn't mean that they're safe and sound. Take a look at the illustration of collaterals for a better idea of what happens inside blocked arteries. We discuss the specific risks associated with elevated LDL levels in the next section.

As cholesterol deposits itself inside an artery, the artery narrows and forms collaterals, or bypasses.

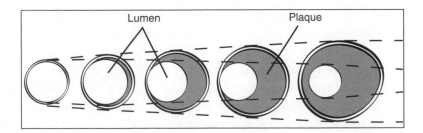

How LDL Increases Health Risks

The main concern with LDL is that it damages the blood vessels and leads to serious health problems. LDL is a major threat to the heart, blood vessels, and all the organs in the body (because they need the heart and blood vessels to provide them with blood). Furthermore, the health risks associated with LDL are linear: the higher the LDL, the greater the risk to a person's health.

Narrowing Things Down

When LDL is deposited in the blood vessels, it can take one several forms. One of its incarnations is called *oxidized LDL*, a highly dangerous manifestation of LDL. In Chapter 1, we talked about cholesterol and inflammation. To summarize that discussion, cholesterol can act as an inflammatory substance, which initiates an attack of specialized cells called macrophages. The macrophages eat the cholesterol and spit out a burst of toxins that damages the blood vessels.

Oxidized LDL pulls inflammatory cells toward it; as a result, it plays a key part in the development of a condition called *atherosclerosis*, or a narrowing of the arteries.

def•i•ni•tion

Oxidized LDL is a particularly dangerous form of LDL. It acts as a magnet and pulls inflammatory cells toward it. The inflammation results in a burst of toxins, which damages blood vessel walls.

Atherosclerosis is a narrowing of the arteries caused by the deposit of cholesterol on the blood vessel wall. In time, the artery can become completely blocked.

LDL, Plaque, and a Heart Attack

Most heart attacks occur in arteries where the cholesterol-laden plaque has reduced the opening inside the vessel by 40 to 60 percent. The narrowing occurs over years or decades, allowing ample time for collaterals (basically, blood detour routes) to form. These collaterals are like baby bean sprout roots that form around the narrowing, maintaining flow. These collaterals act similar to the service road that bypasses the traffic clogging up the Long Island Expressway. The service road maintains flow. People die of heart disease because of a sudden plaque fracture, breakage, or rupture that some form of stress causes (such as a recently smoked cigarette, a fight with a loved one, or some sort of physical strain). This sudden change causes a blood clot to form; the clot obstructs blood flow to the heart muscle or brain tissue (depending on which artery we're talking about). This takes place over a period of seconds to minutes, and there's just not enough time for the arteries to compensate by forming collaterals.

Often, because LDL is a highly inflammatory substance, an elevated LDL puts the cholesterol plaque at an elevated risk for rupturing and leading to a heart attack. For one thing, LDL is an oxidized compound and is toxic to the inner lining of the blood vessels. Oxidized LDL also pulls more inflammatory cells toward it. These cells infiltrate the plaque and destabilize it, which can lead to plaque rupture, a blood clot, and a subsequent heart attack.

Oh, My Aching Legs!

Leg pain is nothing to fool around with. It can be a sign of serious cardiovascular disease, and our nemesis LDL just might be to blame.

When LDL is circulating around the bloodstream looking for a place to settle, it just might find itself coming to rest in the *aorta* and peripheral blood vessels that lead to the legs. This can result in pain while walking, or even while you're sitting perfectly still!

LDL just needs an artery to do damage—and it doesn't need to be an artery anywhere near the heart. We know, for example, that LDL contributes to the development of strokes by depositing itself in the arteries of the neck and brain.

Clotting

When LDL is deposited in the arteries, it leads to an intense inflammatory response that encourages more cholesterol to bind itself to the artery wall. The inflammation increases the risk that of clot formation at the site, which can restrict blood flow through the artery, for one thing. A clot can also break free and lead to a heart attack or stroke.

Sources of LDL

It's easy to elevate your LDL levels. Many common and easily obtained foods can drive up LDL levels rapidly. In fact, it is more difficult to obtain foods that will *not* drive up LDL.

Many foods are laden with hidden fat calories, and this is what causes in increase in LDL levels. Fat is so common in the American diet that more than 30 percent of the American diet is composed of fat! Sources of LDL include fried foods, baked foods, pastries, cookies, cheese, sauces, dairy products, and many types of beef.

We'll talk more about specific types of fat—including which fats are most harmful in terms of LDL production—in the following section.

> **Here's to Your Heart**
>
> Interested in knowing how much saturated fat you're eating? Start keeping a diet journal. You may be surprised to note how many high-fat foods you're consuming over the course of any given time period (a week, a day, a month). These foods are common sources of LDL; avoiding these foods will lower your LDL.

Avoiding LDL

The best way to avoid LDL (and to therefore lower your LDL levels and your risk of serious health issues, such as heart attack and stroke) is to stop eating fattening foods! However, there's a catch. Like cholesterol, we can break fat down into a good type and a bad type. (And I'll tell you right now: the fat you find in your burger drive-through falls into the bad category!)

A Fat Primer

Trying to decipher saturated fats from unsaturated fats can be really confusing. One difference is the amount of hydrogen each type of fat contains.

All fats are composed of long chains of carbon molecules. Hydrogen atoms are attached to the carbon atoms. The more hydrogen that is attached to the carbon chain, the more saturated the molecule of fat is. Each carbon chain can contain a maximum number of hydrogen atoms. When the chains contain the maximum amount of hydrogen atoms, they're referred to as *saturated* (and conversely, when they have fewer than the maximum number of hydrogen atoms, they're *unsaturated*). There are several illustrations of the various types of fat included in this chapter that will help you to visualize and understand the difference between them.

Saturated fat molecule.

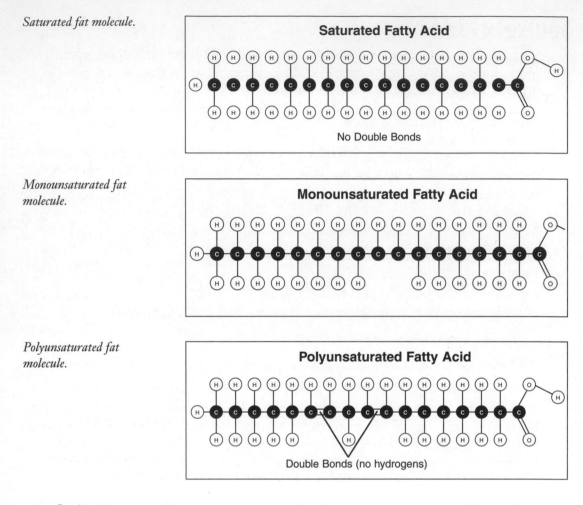

Monounsaturated fat molecule.

Polyunsaturated fat molecule.

So, in summary:

- ◆ **Saturated fats** have the most hydrogen.

- ◆ **Polyunsaturated fats** contain the least hydrogen.

- ◆ **Monounsaturated fats** have one fewer hydrogen atom than saturated fats.

The difference between these various fats lies in where they end up. Saturated fats are converted into LDL particles, whereas polyunsaturated and monounsaturated fats are more likely to be used in the production of HDL, which is the protective cholesterol. When compared side by side, polyunsaturated fat is healthier.

Saturated with Health Risks

Saturated fats are found in highly processed foods, as the processing adds hydrogen atoms to the carbons, thereby saturating them. Scientists did an experiment where they fed lab rats food that was high in saturated fats. Within a short period of time, the rats' LDL levels rose. (So imagine what 20 or 30 years' worth of ingesting saturated fats does to a human!)

A high-fat diet increases LDL levels, while a low-fat diet helps to reduce LDL in the bloodstream. And because even the healthiest diet provides us with all the cholesterol the body needs, there's no need for us to look for some sort of cholesterol supplement, such as onion rings or whole milk. That's courting disaster!

Foods that are high in saturated fats include ...

◆ Fried foods

◆ High-fat dairy foods (ice cream, cheese, whole milk)

◆ High-fat animal meats (such as veal, poultry skin, lamb, and pork)

◆ Baked goods and pastries

◆ Foods processed with palm oil (these can vary—microwave popcorn may contain palm oil, and your morning coffee may, too)

Saturated fats cause damage to the cells on the inside of the arteries, or endothelial cells. They can also cause an inflammatory effect on the inside of the blood vessels, resulting in a greater degree of plaque formation. The excess inflammation is responsible for a greater likelihood of plaque rupture and subsequent heart attack.

Polyunsaturated Fat

Some fats, called *polyunsaturated fats*, are actually beneficial to health because they work to reduce cholesterol levels. Polyunsaturated fats can be found in foods such as ...

◆ Vegetable oils

◆ Most nuts

◆ Olives

◆ Avocados

◆ Salmon

A diet rich in polyunsaturated fats can actually lower LDL and the risk of cardiac disease. In Part 2 of this book, we discuss heart-healthy nutrition in more detail.

Here's to Your Heart _____

Education, moderation and common sense are the keys to a healthy lifestyle, especially where diet is concerned. Healthy eating comes down to making the healthiest possible food choices, and you can't do this if you don't know which foods are healthy and which are unhealthy. Some types of fat are more acceptable than others, for example. It's healthier for you to have a handful of nuts than to eat a big slab of cake. The nuts contain polyunsaturated fat, which can lower LDL; the cake contains saturated fat, which raises cholesterol levels. We'll talk more about choosing healthy foods in Part 2 of this book.

The Least You Need to Know

◆ LDL stands for low-density lipoprotein; it is the "bad" or harmful type of cholesterol.

◆ The liver converts fat into LDL.

◆ Newborns have LDL levels of 25–40 mg/dl; the average adult LDL level is between 130 and 160 mg/dl.

◆ Saturated fats are easily converted in LDL; polyunsaturated and monounsaturated fats are more likely to wind up as HDL in the bloodstream.

Chapter **3**

HDL: The Good Cholesterol

In This Chapter

◆ Learn about the protective nature of HDL

◆ Understand why it's important to raise your HDL levels

◆ Discover ways to lower LDL and raise HDL at the same time

◆ Get a feel for how HDL is broken down into even smaller elements

◆ See what the future holds for HDL-enhancing techniques

We discussed the dark side of cholesterol in Chapter 2. Now we're going to turn the page, both literally and figuratively, and talk about some of cholesterol's redeeming qualities.

In contrast to the grim reality and adversity posed by LDL, *HDL*, or *high density lipoprotein*, is a relatively protective component of cholesterol. The role of HDL is to *remove* cholesterol from inside the blood vessels. Because HDL is such a good Roto-Rooter in this sense, one of the primary goals of modifying your cholesterol levels is to raise HDL levels. In this chapter, we talk about what HDL is, why cardiologists prefer to see high HDL numbers (as opposed to elevated LDL levels), and various methods used to raise HDL.

What Is HDL?

In Chapter 1, we talked about a lab test called centrifuge. This is where a vial of blood is taken and spun 'round and 'round to separate the various components of the blood (such as platelets, red blood cells, and white blood cells).

def•i•ni•tion

HDL stands for **high-density lipoprotein**. HDL is believed to play a protective role in the bloodstream, cleaning up the plaque that LDL leaves behind.

Centrifuging blood removes the cells that float around in the blood. What's left over is a material called plasma, which is essentially the blood minus the cells. Plasma can be further centrifuged down to yield creamy supernatant (the liquid that's left when everything else has been spun out) that contains the various cholesterol subfractions. The subfractions closest to the top of the cream are the lightest, or least dense, such as LDL. The highest density components, such as HDL, are at the bottom of the cream.

For men, the goal is to raise HDL to greater than 40 mg/dl. For women, the goal is to raise HDL to greater than 50 mg/dl. An *ideal* HDL level is anything above 60 mg/dl. An HDL below 40 mg/dl confers increased risk of heart attack and stroke. In people who have other risk factors (such as tobacco smoking, obesity, and diabetes) the impetus to raise HDL is stronger because low HDL becomes a more powerful risk factor when combined with concomitant risks.

The Many Faces of HDL

HDL is composed of smaller parts called subfractions: HDL2 and HDL3. Though these components are still the subject of intense study at this moment, it is believed that HDL2 might be the protective component of HDL, whereas HDL3 is believed to offer less protection against elevated LDL levels.

Diet, exercise, alcohol in moderation, and medication may work to increase the HDL2 component. Interestingly, when people eat high-fat diets, their HDL may increase, along with their LDL and total cholesterol levels. But even though the HDL levels increase, these individuals may not obtain the protection of an elevated HDL because it is believed that the HDL that's on the rise is HDL3—the less protective subfraction.

Healthy Heart Facts

Another interesting property of HDL is the apparent strength of its risk in the context of heart trouble. Often, a person will come to the hospital with a heart attack and have a cholesterol panel drawn at the time of admission. We find that this person has an adequately low LDL (under 100), but further exploration will demonstrate an isolated low HDL. *This may be the single most important risk factor responsible for the heart attack.*

APO A

Like other cholesterol that floats around in the bloodstream, HDL consists of a central cholesterol core surrounded by a protein coat. However, the protein coat that surrounds HDL is different than the protein that's wrapped around LDL. HDL's protein coat goes by the name of *APO A*.

What's so great about this APO A? Is it some sort of cholesterol superhero? Is it a miracle-working protein? Can it go where no cholesterol has gone before? APO A does your body a lot of good. It allows HDL to bind to an area of a blood vessel wall that needs a blast of cholesterol-reducing power. Imagine a pipe that's caked with gunk. You pour in some drain cleaner, and the gunk slips away. APO A works in a similar way, clearing the blood vessels of potentially life-threatening cholesterol gunk.

def•i•ni•tion _____

APO A is the name given to the protein that coats HDL, or the good cholesterol. APO A facilitates the removal of harmful cholesterol in the blood vessels.

Why Raise HDL?

You want to raise HDL levels as high as possible to achieve optimum health. Back in Chapter 2, we talked about the negative effects of LDL, including an increased risk of heart attack and stroke, and a general decline in health. Every single blood vessel in your body affects your overall health; if your blood vessels are clogged with cholesterol, you're not going to be doing so well (at least not in the long run).

Chapter 2 also talked about how LDL encourages the formation of plaque inside blood vessels. HDL helps the body to rid itself of the cholesterol contained in plaque. And after the cholesterol is removed, the plaque becomes more stable and less likely to rupture when subjected to various stressors. This, in turn, means that clot formation over the plaque is less likely. Ultimately this means that the risk of heart attack and stroke is also reduced.

What HDL Does for Your Arteries

HDL does for your arteries what your vacuum cleaner does for your living room rug (*after* you've let the kids run wild in there with snacks and crafts and friends and the dog). After years of living the high life, feasting on high-fat snacks and meals, your arteries may be a mess. You've got LDL and plaque clinging to the walls, and you may even be feeling some of the effects of having unhealthy arteries (leg pain, for example, or chest pain).

Here comes HDL to clean up some of the mess: it swooshes through your arteries, looking for bad cholesterol to bind itself to. After it meets up with its nemesis, it forces the bad cholesterol to give up its grip on your blood vessel wall (and, by extension, on your health), and HDL whisks the bad stuff away. Your arteries look a whole lot better, and your health improves as a result.

If HDL could talk, it would tell you that no thanks is necessary. It's just doing its job.

How HDL Protects Your Health

Generally speaking, HDL is protective and reduces the risk of heart disease. Simply put, people who have high levels of HDL have a lower risk for developing heart attack and stroke. It's natural that you'd want to know more about this wondrous component of cholesterol. Well, most doctors feel the same way.

The truth is, the data supporting HDL as a force for LDL to reckon with is not as strong as the scientific evidence that tells us that LDL is bad for us. We do know, however, that people who have elevated HDL levels tend to be healthier than those who have elevated LDL levels, and that they tend to have fewer heart attacks and strokes. Ideally, then, it's in your best interest to lower LDL as much as possible while simultaneously working to raise HDL levels.

What's Good for LDL Is Great for HDL

In general, it's much more difficult to raise HDL levels than it is to lower LDL levels. In one sense, that's fine. Because LDL is so harmful to your health, you want to lower it, after all. But in another sense, this news is disheartening, because we know that a person with an average LDL level and a low HDL level can still be at risk for serious health problems. It's fine and well (and essential, by the way) to drop that LDL, but it may not always be enough to prevent heart attack and stroke.

Here's a piece of good news, though: interventions that lower LDL tend to raise HDL at the same time. For example …

- ◆ If you're cutting back on fried foods and eating a low-fat diet rich in fruits and vegetables, you're killing two birds with one stone.

- ◆ Exercise lowers your bad cholesterol while encouraging your good cholesterol levels to climb, and it may be one of the most effective ways to elevate HDL levels.

- ◆ Medications that work to suppress LDL levels simultaneously raise HDL levels.

Again, though, it's just not as easy to raise HDL as it is to lower LDL.

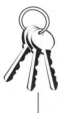

Here's to Your Heart _____

Elevating HDL levels is kind of like the graduate school of cholesterol modification. Like having a four-year degree from college, lowering your LDL will only get you so far. To shoot past the other candidates who are in line for a job (or, in this case, better health), you've got to be dedicated and willing to work *that much* harder to achieve your goals. It's not necessarily impossible; it just takes a lot of determination and effort.

You should strive to follow the guidelines for LDL and HDL levels. The important thing to remember, though, is that these guidelines are fairly conservative—that is, you can always go lower with your LDL and higher with your HDL, no matter where your numbers happen to be in relation to the guidelines. The current recommendations for cholesterol levels are under scrutiny by the medical community. Chances are, we'll see some modifications of those numbers (recommendations for even lower LDL levels and higher HDL levels) sometime in the not-so-distant future.

HDL and Alcohol

The role alcohol plays in mitigating heart disease is somewhat controversial. Studies have noted that men who consume one to two drinks per day and women who consume one drink per day have a decreased risk of heart attack and stroke. Researchers studied large groups of people who consumed alcohol in moderation on a daily basis. These people were observed to have a lower incidence of heart disease. Part of this may be due to an elevation of HDL (specifically HDL2) by alcohol.

The Doctor Says _____

To achieve alcohol-related HDL elevations, it probably doesn't matter what type of alcohol you drink, because the benefit seems to be equal with all types. There may be a red wine–specific benefit related to antioxidants and other compounds in red wine, but this is still up for debate in the medical community. Some of alcohol's protective effects may be due to other factors besides elevating HDL, although this is not currently known.

Though this may be contrary to what your pals are telling you, doctors *do not* suggest that their patients start drinking. (And insurance companies have no intention of instituting a wine-coverage policy.) However, men and women who already consume a drink or two each day need not stop (unless there are other health issues that would make it necessary for them to discontinue this practice). And here's a piece of information that's important: consuming more than the recommended one to two drinks per day leads to an *increased risk* for heart disease! The old adage "Everything in moderation" certainly holds true here.

Sources and Resources for HDL

Wouldn't it be great if you could pop into a health food store, sidle up to the counter, and say, "I'll take some powdered HDL. How much is that, about $8 a pound?" Cardiologists everywhere would hand out coupons ("$1 off HDL next Thursday!") instead of prescriptions.

Unfortunately it doesn't work that way. You can't buy HDL at the store, pick it from trees, or grow it in the ground. In fact, there really aren't any sources of HDL in the diet, which is one reason it's not as easy to raise HDL levels as it is to lower LDL levels. If you recall, lowering LDL levels requires modifications to diet and exercise. Sometimes, a person will need medication to help lower LDL. Modifying HDL levels is far more complex.

Even though HDL isn't contained in food per se (that is, you can't grab a particular snack, read the nutrition label, and pick out one ingredient that contains HDL), there are some foods that help the body to produce HDL. Some of the best dietary boosters for HDL levels include ...

Healthy Heart Facts

HDL is a by-product of complex metabolic processes in the body that facilitate conversion of one type of cholesterol to another. Although the heart benefits from this conversion, the liver also plays a major role in this process.

- Olive oil

- Canola oil

- Soy and flaxseed oils

- Nuts, such as almonds, peanuts, pecans, and cashews

- Coldwater fish, such as salmon and mackerel

Foods that are rich in processed, complex carbohydrates, such as breads and cereals, will also tend to elevate HDL.

> **Healthy Heart Facts**
>
> While nuts and other unsaturated fats can help to raise HDL levels, moderation is always the key to a healthy diet. The goal is to replace saturated fats in your diet (the vegetable oil you normally cook with, for example) with unsaturated fats (like olive oil). We'll talk more about fat in Chapter 4, and in Chapter 8 we'll talk about functional foods (foods that help to improve your health).

Move It and Raise It

Exercise is a good way to stimulate HDL production; however, the overall increase in HDL may only amount to about 5 percent. This doesn't sound like a significant number, but remember, any increase in HDL is beneficial. Plus, as previously mentioned, when HDL rises, that usually means that LDL is on the downswing. In with the good and out with the bad.

We don't really know *how* HDL is raised through aerobic exercise, but we do know that the primary benefit comes from about 30 minutes of aerobic exercise a day, at least five days a week. The American Heart Association suggests that the *total* duration of daily aerobic activity be equal to or greater than 30 minutes per day. This is good news for those of you who hate to break a sweat: those 30 minutes can be divided into smaller increments throughout the course of the day! So really, there's no good excuse *not* to get your body moving.

Here's to Your Heart

A decrease in LDL because of exercise might cause a shift in the ratio of HDL to LDL. This shift may just be more beneficial to health than the percentage of increase of HDL. In other words, as long as HDL is increasing and suppressing LDL, the *rate* of increase isn't what we're concerned with.

Benefits of Pumping Up Your HDL

Interestingly, your cardiac risk is reduced about 3 percent for every 1 percent increase in HDL. Meanwhile, for every 1 percent reduction in LDL, the risk reduction is 2 percent. In short, raising your HDL levels does more to decrease your risk of heart trouble than *only* lowering your LDL.

Even when you institute several methods—such as diet, exercise, and medication—to raise HDL, the elevation may only total 5 percent or so. This increase, even though it seems minor and limited (especially when you consider how much effort you've put into modifying your diet, exercise, and medications), can actually be quite significant. When HDL levels are increased, the risk reduction for heart disease is 1 percent to 2 percent. And as I said earlier in this chapter, for a 1 percent reduction in LDL, a 2 percent reduction in cardiovascular risk is achieved. Therefore, seemingly minor elevations in HDL are actually quite significant and powerful.

Little Helpers

Recently some physicians have begun to measure HDL subfractions. There are at least two significant varieties of HDL: HDL2 and HDL3. It is believed that HDL2 is protective, whereas HDL3 is less protective. Interventions that target HDL elevation (such as diet, exercise, and medication) and decrease cardiac risk do so by elevating HDL2. HDL subfraction measurement is not universal, however. Much of the work done in the study of HDL subfractions is still experimental.

In the future, HDL may commonly be considered in terms of the ratios between HDL subfractions. For example, cholesterol reduction through a low-fat diet may reduce the total cholesterol, including HDL. If you've been paying attention, you know that we want HDL to *increase*, so this may sound like bad news. However, this decrease in HDL may not be a negative thing, because it could mean that there's been a drop in HDL3, which is the less protective element of HDL.

HDL Italiano

When people consume low-fat diets, their HDL levels may decrease along with their LDL and total cholesterol levels. Although their HDL levels decrease, the ratio of HDL2 to HDL3 may become more favorable and, therefore, more protective. This phenomenon of a low, yet protective HDL is best exemplified by the HDL Milano variant. Researchers noted that a certain Italian population had low levels of HDL, yet a low incidence of heart disease. It became apparent that despite a low HDL, these people were protected by a variant of HDL (in other words, they had high levels of HDL2, which, again, is the protective element of HDL) that was super-efficient at removing cholesterol.

Healthy Heart Facts

HDL2 is being examined for its potential ability to "vacuum clean" the inside of the arteries. In fact, researchers are exploring the possibility of infusing HDL into the bloodstream of a person who is having a heart attack in order to reduce clotting by cleaning the inside of arteries and reversing the damage of many years of dietary indiscretion and elevated LDL. These exciting experiments may revolutionize the treatment of cholesterol disorders and, therefore, of heart disease.

The end result of Milano study was the understanding that there are ways to amplify, or increase, the effects of HDL by increasing its levels and/or its protective subfractions (like HDL2) dramatically, and we should be working toward finding *more* ways to do this. Drugs that act like HDL are being studied in heart attack patients to reduce the amount of cholesterol inside the arteries. This rapid reduction of cholesterol may reduce the risk of death in these patients.

For example, cardiologists use a class of medications called CETP inhibitors, which elevate HDL and allow HDL to remove cholesterol from inside the arteries. Future research is aimed at determining whether CETP inhibitors and other interventions to dramatically raise HDL levels will reduce death from heart disease and stroke. For most doctors, however, the evidence is clear enough already: we advise patients to raise their HDL levels. We discuss CETP inhibitors in more detail in Chapter 23. At this time, because HDL is so difficult to control at our own will, the focus is mainly on reducing LDL.

Healthy Heart Facts

Recent evidence suggests that after a heart attack, CETP inhibitors can be infused into the bloodstream and rapidly remove deposited cholesterol from the inside of blood vessels. This is very exciting since these drugs may reverse years, if not decades, of chronic damage over a very short period of time (days or weeks).

The Least You Need to Know

◆ HDL is composed of the subfractions HDL2 and HDL3.

◆ It is believed that HDL3 plays a role in protecting the blood vessels from elevated LDL levels.

- One to two alcoholic drinks per day may help to stimulate HDL levels.

- Just 30 minutes of aerobic exercise a day, five days a week is a good way to raise HDL levels.

- Just about any intervention that works to lower LDL levels will also raise LDL levels and affect the ratio of HDL to LDL in the bloodstream.

Understanding Triglycerides

In This Chapter

- Understand the difference between triglycerides and cholesterol
- Discover the true purpose of triglycerides and what happens when their levels in the body become too high
- Know how triglycerides affect the blood vessels
- Make the link between triglycerides and diabetes
- Learn how to control your triglyceride levels and simultaneously drop your LDL and raise your HDL

When you go for a cholesterol screening, you'll no doubt also get a report about your triglyceride levels. Many people take this news in stride, figuring that because the doctor took the time to order this test that it must have some relation to cholesterol and heart health. But do you really know what triglycerides are, where they come from, or (perhaps most importantly) what they mean to your overall well-being?

We know far more about the effect of LDL and HDL on health than we know about triglycerides. However, there is little doubt that these fatty components of the blood can lead to serious health issues, especially if someone has high triglyceride levels *and* a preexisting condition, such as obesity or diabetes. In this chapter we define triglycerides, and discuss what they do to your body and how you can work to lower them to acceptable levels.

What Are Triglycerides?

Triglycerides are fatty compounds that circulate in the blood, just like HDL and LDL. However, the chemical structure of triglycerides differs from LDL, HDL, and other cholesterol subfractions, and this is what makes triglycerides unique among the fats in your bloodstream.

Comparing Cholesterol and Triglycerides

In Chapter 1, we talked about how cholesterol is needed and where it is utilized by the body. Cholesterol is essentially a steroid compound. The chemical makeup of steroids allows them to be used by cells to build other compounds. One of cholesterol's functions is in the production of the male and female hormones.

def•i•ni•tion

Triglycerides are fatty substances that circulate in the bloodstream. Although triglycerides are routinely measured in a cholesterol panel, their chemical makeup and basic functions differ from cholesterol.

Triglycerides, meanwhile, are made up of an alcohol called *glycerol* with three long carbon chains of variable lengths attached, although sometimes only two chains will attach themselves. When only two chains are attached, the third site can accommodate a different molecule. The molecule that attaches to this third site is incredibly important, because it determines how the body will use the substance that is formed here.

For example, one type of triglyceride compound has a glycerol (alcohol) backbone, and two long fatty chains; at that third site, a molecule called a phospholipid is attached. One place that phospholipid-based glycerols can be found is in the sheaths that cover our nerves. If a different type of molecule attached itself to that site, the entire triglyceride compound would be used elsewhere in the body.

A Fat Recap

The roles of various long fatty chains are determined by the number of carbons in the chains and the number of hydrogen atoms that surround each carbon atom. If this discussion sounds vaguely familiar, it should. We discussed the formation of fat in Chapter 2.

To review:

♦ When each carbon atom is surrounded by the maximum number of hydrogen atoms, the fatty chain is called *saturated*.

♦ If a carbon atom binds only one hydrogen atom, it is *unsaturated*.

♦ If many carbons in the chain are accompanied by only one hydrogen item, it is *polyunsaturated*.

♦ A *monounsaturated* compound has only one carbon accompanied by a single hydrogen atom.

Remember, poly- and monounsaturated fats are more likely to be used in the production of HDL, the protective cholesterol.

The fatty chains that contribute to elevated LDL are all saturated with the maximum number of carbon atoms. Their names are *lauric acid*, *myristic acid*, and *palmitic acid*. These fatty chains are called *fatty acids*, and are commonly found in dairy, meat, and tropical oils (such as palm and coconut). They form part of the core of the LDL packages, which causes damage to the arteries(as they are part of the cholesterol plaque that occludes arteries).

In contrast, there are other fatty acid chains that are relatively healthy. One such type of fatty acid is called oleic acid, which is *monounsaturated*. Oleic acid can be found in canola and olive oil. Another healthy fatty acid is called linoleic acid. Linoleic acid also has 18 carbons, two of which have only one hydrogen atom per carbon atom. This is a *polyunsaturated* fatty acid. It can be found in seed and vegetable oils such as safflower, sunflower, and corn oils.

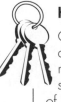

Here's to Your Heart

Canola and olive oils comprise a major portion of the Mediterranean type diet, which was shown to reduce the incidence of heart disease in a major study called the Lyon Heart Study. We talk about the Mediterranean diet in more detail in Chapter 7.

Burger In, Triglycerides Up

Here's what's so dangerous about triglyceride levels: after you eat any meal (fatty or not), triglycerides will *immediately* increase in the bloodstream (and recede later). After eating a meal that's loaded with fat (like your average trip to your favorite fast food restaurant), triglycerides levels experience an extreme surge. Doctors are particularly concerned with this type of elevation in triglyceride levels, because it may do immediate harm to the blood vessels. Triglycerides can be deposited as plaque, which, as you know by now, harms the arteries because it prevents them from performing their basic function of dilating and allowing blood to flow freely.

Here's something interesting that really illustrates the negative power of triglycerides: doctors now have a machine that measures the health of the blood vessels. (It's a device that measures how "springy" a blood vessel is.) When a tourniquet is wrapped around the arm, blood flow stops. When the tourniquet is released, the arteries dilate rapidly and allow a surge of blood to flow. A young, healthy, physically fit individual who consumes a low-fat diet will likely have springy arteries that dilate rapidly after the tourniquet is released. However, if this same person has this test done within an hour after a fattening meal (laden with triglycerides and saturated fat), he would see an acute decrease in the blood vessel springiness.

The decrease in springiness is due to acute injury to the blood vessels! Triglycerides can cause quick and certain harm to the blood vessels, which makes them less able to dilate and allow blood to circulate to areas where it is needed.

The Doctor Says

The rise in triglycerides following a high-fat meal may acutely damage the inner lining of the blood vessels. For this reason, it's believed that triglycerides may be pro-atherogenic, which is to say that they contribute additional plaque buildup in the blood vessels.

Most of us like to believe that any harm that fat does to our bodies is done over the long term. We know, for example, that cholesterol accumulates and does most of its damage over a period of years or decades. This is not the case with triglycerides. Though they aren't discussed quite as often as cholesterol is, they can do quite a bit of damage in a short period of time.

How Triglycerides Harm Your Health

The cause-and-effect link between triglycerides and heart disease has been more difficult to establish than the link between elevated cholesterol levels and heart disease. There are some disorders, such as pancreatic disease, thyroid disorders, and various hormone disorders, that are characterized by high levels of triglycerides; however, these disorders don't carry an increased risk of heart attack and stroke. Conversely, there are some conditions, such as type 2 diabetes, that are characterized by modest elevations in triglycerides, but have a strong link to heart disease.

When it's put that way, it sounds like triglycerides are perhaps nothing for the heart to fear, right? Well, let's not go that far. Although it was once believed that elevated triglyceride levels were a risk factor for heart disease only if they teamed up with low

HDL levels, recent evidence suggests triglycerides play an independent role in the development of heart disease.

So even though scientists might be missing a definitive link or two in these studies, they have good reason to believe that elevated triglycerides *are* harmful. Elevated triglycerides are also most often noted with abnormal levels of other cholesterol subfractions: typically, elevated triglycerides occur in a person who also has high LDL levels and low HDL levels. Diabetics often present all three abnormalities in their cholesterol panel. And, as you know by now, this is a dangerous, dangerous combination.

> **Healthy Heart Facts**
>
> Various metabolic disorders may also cause a triglyceride level to become elevated. Hypothyroidism is one such disorder, and some diseases of the liver can also affect triglycerides. Although these problems begin in the metabolic system, they can wind up affecting the health of one's cardiovascular system.

Metabolic Syndrome and Heart Health

Elevated triglycerides are often seen in a condition called *metabolic syndrome*, which is a highly prevalent disorder in affluent countries (such as the United States and the countries of Western Europe). Metabolic syndrome is essentially a by-product of the typical American lifestyle: eating a diet that's high in fat and leading a sedentary lifestyle. This is why this disorder is mainly seen in affluent regions; you just don't see a lot of Africans or Eskimos, for example, sitting around stuffing themselves with fast food while watching TV on a regular basis.

def•i•ni•tion

> **Metabolic syndrome** refers to a group of health issues that raise a person's risk for developing heart attack and stroke. Elevated triglycerides are one element of the metabolic syndrome.

Obesity is diagnosed when a person has a *BMI, or body mass index,* of over 30; a person is considered overweight when his BMI is between 25 and 29.9. Obesity is becoming a common (and serious) health issue in this country. Therefore, because being overweight or obese plays a role in developing metabolic syndrome, you probably actually know someone who either has metabolic syndrome or is headed in that direction. In fact, it's estimated that 25 percent of the people in the United States may have metabolic syndrome, and unfortunately, it's becoming more and more common in children and adolescents.

What's so bad about metabolic syndrome? It sounds like it might jump-start your metabolism, which, actually, doesn't sound like a bad deal at all. Needless to say, a high metabolism is *not* the hallmark symptom of metabolic syndrome. There are several different definitions for metabolic syndrome utilizing various criteria, but they all have several key factors in common. In addition to having elevated triglycerides, people who have metabolic syndrome ...

◆ Are above their ideal body weight.

◆ Have an elevated systolic blood pressure (the top number in a blood pressure reading).

◆ Lead a sedentary lifestyle.

◆ Have a large abdominal girth (40 inches or more for men; 36 inches or more for women).

◆ May have diabetes mellitus (also called type 2 diabetes).

◆ Have elevated LDL levels and low HDL levels.

Take another look at this list. What do all of these factors have in common? The symptoms of metabolic syndrome are basically risk factors for heart disease. When all these elements work together, the risk for developing heart attack and stroke is alarmingly high.

Here's to Your Heart

Being overweight or obese can lead to developing many risk factors for heart disease and stroke. How do doctors determine if someone is over their ideal weight? They use the **body mass index,** or **BMI,** to measure a patient's degree of adiposity (or, in lay terms, just how overweight someone is). We measure a person's BMI by dividing height in meters by body weight in kilograms squared. An acceptable body mass is approximately 25 kg/m2 (or lower). An obese body mass comes out at about 30 kg/m2. An overweight body mass can fall between these two measurements.

Diabetes and Triglycerides

Obese patients typically have several *lipid* subfraction abnormalities, such as an elevation of LDL elevations, a low level of HDL, and elevated triglycerides.

In addition, obese patients often have a condition called *insulin resistance*, which is basically a prediabetic state. (Unless some drastic changes in health take place, this person is going to be a diabetic in the near future.) And after someone develops diabetes, they're predisposed to elevated triglycerides.

Why does this happen? What does elevated blood sugar have to do with elevated triglycerides? Sure, sugar and fat are a couple of substances that shouldn't be floating around in excess in the bloodstream, but they're still two separate entities, so what's the deal here? Does sugar magically transform itself into fat or what? As humans deposit fat around their waistlines, their blood sugars tend to rise (which is why being obese or merely being significantly overweight is a risk factor for developing diabetes). But even before blood sugar levels start to rise, there may already be years of insulin resistance at work, and the body may already be worn down by trying to fight a losing battle.

> **Healthy Heart Facts**
>
> **Lipid** is a synonym for fat. When we talk about lipid subfractions, we're talking about the various fatty substances that are floating around in the bloodstream, such as HDL, LDL, and triglycerides. A cholesterol panel *is* a lipid panel—it measures the fat circulating in the blood.

def•i•ni•tion

> In every body, the pancreas secretes insulin to metabolize glucose, or sugar. If someone's insulin is no longer able to metabolize glucose the way that it should, you call this condition **insulin resistance**. The problem lies with the receptors on the muscle cell membranes that become resistant to insulin or less responsive. This results in more insulin being required to maintain a normal blood sugar. The result is elevated blood sugar after eating. Insulin resistance can lead to diabetes, which in turn leads to elevated triglyceride levels.

Before someone develops full-blown diabetes, blood sugar creeps up. It will be high at times when it is supposed to be normal. Often, it will *only* be at the high end of normal, or remain high after eating longer than it should. The sugar oxidizes protein in the body, which causes damage to the internal organs. This damage brings in inflammatory cells, which is described earlier. These inflammatory cells cause further damage and eventually cause blood clots, heart attacks, and strokes.

Diabetes is preceded by obesity 90 percent of the time. (Maybe only 10 percent of diabetics are skinny, and these people usually have some other problem, such as a mutation that affects the pancreas's ability to make insulin.) Abdominal fat, in particular, is really dangerous. Belly fat is metabolically different from, say thigh or gluteal (rear-end) fat. (You can think of this as an "apple-shaped" body being more unhealthy than a "pear-shaped" body.) Fat that settles around the waist produces some harmful substances that cause inflammation and clotting and also contributes to the development of diabetes. We can say, then, that abdominal fat is pro-diabetic and pro-atherogenic.

The Doctor Says

> The sugar damages the blood vessels all over the body: the eyes are affected, and so are the feet, kidneys, brain heart—all the organs. This leads to early vision loss and amputations, as well as infections (because of poor blood supply). In fact, diabetes is the leading cause of preventable blindness and amputations in the United States.

Understanding Triglyceride Levels

When you're thinking about your triglyceride level, you need to take other factors into consideration. Everything's relative, even when it comes to your lipid subfractions. (That would make a nice bumper-sticker mantra, wouldn't it?) It's important to read triglyceride levels in context, because, as I said at the beginning of the chapter, a fatty meal can cause a spike in triglycerides. That alone doesn't necessarily indicate that a person is in grave danger of developing heart disease…but taken with other factors, it could.

Ideally, triglycerides should be no higher than 150 mg/dl. Levels above 400 mg/dl can be particularly dangerous.

Look At the Bigger Picture

Elevated triglycerides are more serious in the presence of elevated LDL and low HDL levels. And, as we just discussed in the previous section, an elevated triglyceride level coupled with insulin resistance or diabetes can cause dire health problems. The body is breaking down on several levels at that point; the risk for heart attack and stroke are greatly magnified as compared to someone who has an elevated triglyceride level but whose blood sugar remains at normal levels. The prediabetic has the added misfortune of the bloodstream working to convert sugar into fat.

Frequently elevated triglycerides are in the context of other disorders, such as hypothyroidism and liver disease. Obviously, these secondary causes of raised triglycerides need to be corrected before the triglycerides can be treated via medication.

Healthy Heart Facts
Interestingly, the use of oral contraceptives can also result in elevated triglyceride levels. If you're using some sort of oral contraceptive, or any medication for that matter, make sure your doctor knows about it and notes it in your medical file. Many drugs can cause abnormal blood test results.

Lowering Triglycerides

The previous chapter discussed that working to lower your LDL levels will serve a dual purpose, because your HDL levels will also respond to your efforts. And even if the HDL levels don't shoot up astronomically, you'll affect the ratio of HDL to LDL in the bloodstream, which reduces your risk for developing heart attacks and strokes.

There is even better news now: if you're working to lower your LDL levels and raise your HDL levels, you're likely to see a reduction in your triglyceride levels as well. (That's like killing *three* birds with one stone!) To shift the balance and make HDL the King of the Bloodstream, follow these suggestions:

◆ **Eat a healthy diet.** Foods low in saturated fats, such as fresh fruits and vegetables and low-fat meats (white poultry meat and salmon are good choices).

◆ **Exercise.** Thirty minutes of moderate activity a day, and it doesn't even need to be 30 consecutive minutes. Just get moving somehow, someway, and you'll help your heart's health.

◆ **Take your medications.** Your doctor will tell you whether you're a candidate for triglyceride-lowering meds. If you are, follow your doctor's orders and *take the medicine*.

When more than one abnormal cholesterol subfraction (high LDL, low HDL, high triglycerides) exists in the bloodstream, the effects are synergistic. In other words, these elements work together and feed off one another in a kind of perfect storm of fatty blood elements and greatly magnify the risk of developing a heart attack or stroke. That's why it is so important to address each of these issues as soon as possible, so that the damage can be stopped and hopefully even corrected.

The Least You Need to Know

- Triglycerides are lipids, or fatty substances, circulating in the bloodstream.

- Triglycerides are converted into fatty acids in the body from saturated fats commonly found in foods, such as dairy, high-fat meats, and tropical oils (for example, palm and coconut).

- The blood vessels' ability to dilate is immediately affected after a meal that's loaded with triglycerides.

- Elevated triglycerides play a role in metabolic syndrome, which refers to a group of risk factors for developing heart disease.

- People who have diabetes or who are obese and have high levels of triglycerides are at higher risk of developing heart disease.

Chapter 5

Understanding Risk Factors

In This Chapter

- ◆ Learn about risk factors and how they affect your health
- ◆ Understand the difference between modifiable and unmodifiable risk factors
- ◆ Find ways to improve your health by making small changes to your diet
- ◆ Read the latest recommendations to lower cholesterol
- ◆ Understand how your doctor determines your risk factor score

Can you do anything to prevent your chances of developing heart disease or stroke, either right now or in the future? To determine the likelihood of someone developing an illness, doctors take a look at several different contributing factors. These may include family history, diet, activity level, and age. This chapter explains each of these factors, along with what they mean to you and your risk of developing heart disease or stroke. You will also discover ways that you can change some of these factors and decrease your chances of becoming ill.

What Are Risk Factors?

The likelihood of a person developing an illness is determined by various *risk factors*. There are actually many risk factors for many different diseases. Some might cause disease, and although others may not be directly involved in the development of the disease, they might contribute to an illness developing later in life.

def•i•ni•tion

Risk factors are behaviors, lifestyles, or other factors that increase a person's likelihood of developing a disease or condition. For example, smoking is a risk factor for lung cancer, whereas direct exposure to ultra-violet rays is a risk factor for developing skin cancer. We'll discuss the various risk factors for developing heart disease and stroke throughout this chapter.

Because the link between risk factors and illness isn't always clear, physicians sometimes struggle with definitively saying that a certain lifestyle (or environment or inherited trait) causes a specific condition. For example, until the mid-1980s, there was a dispute in the medical community as to whether elevated levels of cholesterol caused heart disease. (And on a related note, there was, of course, another ongoing debate about whether reducing cholesterol levels were an effective means to prevent heart disease.)

In the past 20 years, numerous studies have positively shown that there is, indeed, a link between elevated cholesterol levels and an increased risk of heart attack and stroke. Likewise, studies have also proved that reducing cholesterol can prevent these conditions. In fact, we now know that the higher the risk for stroke or heart attack, the greater the benefits of reducing cholesterol.

So how do doctors determine who's at risk for heart disease and stroke? It's simple; the greater the number and severity of risk factors a person has for developing these conditions, the greater the threat to that person's health. And as this threat grows, it becomes even more important to drive down that cholesterol level. By modifying or minimizing risk factors, it's possible to lower cholesterol levels and improve a person's overall health.

Sounds easy enough, right? Make some changes to your lifestyle and reap the benefits? Here's the catch: some risk factors can't be modified. There's not much that any of us can do about these specific conditions except to do our best to minimize their effects.

Let's take a look at some of the common risk factors associated with heart disease and stroke. We'll start with the bad news first—those unmodifiable risk factors that you can't change.

Risk Factors You Can't Change

You're a real go-getter and you think that you'll do whatever it takes to modify your risk factors for heart disease and stroke. You live by the motto, "There is nothing I can't do," and you're completely confident that not only can you reduce your risk factors ... heck, you're going to get rid of them altogether!

You're a cardiologist's dream patient, but try as you might, you can't go back in time and erase your family's medical history, your age, and your gender. These are the major unmodifiable risk factors that are covered in this section.

Family History

Your family has handed you a legacy you'd rather not have, one of heart attack and stroke. Family history is a powerful risk factor; it's a cocktail of genetics and environment. Mixing bad genetics with bad eating habits (think grease, grease, and more grease) and a sedentary lifestyle, or a lifestyle including very little physical activity, is a recipe for disaster.

Family history becomes more important as the number of close relatives who have developed a condition or illness increases. For example, a 40-year-old male whose father and brother had heart attacks in their forties is at high risk for having a heart attack himself.

Someone who finds himself in this situation can curse the gene pool he was born into or he can acknowledge that the one thing he can control and change is his lifestyle. In fact, a strong unmodifiable family history can be—and should be—a powerful impetus for getting oneself on the right track and altering the risk factors that *can* be changed. (We'll talk more about modifiable risk factors later in this chapter.)

Healthy Heart Facts

It's well-known that the Japanese have low cholesterol levels and a low incidence of heart disease. Some of this protection comes from having a defensive genetic makeup, at least as far as these conditions are concerned. Interestingly, back in the 1970s, the Ni-Han-San study took a look at the health of Japanese immigrants in Hawaii and San Francisco. The results showed that the Japanese had who immigrated to the continental United States had developed an increased risk of heart disease—an example of genetic modification going in the wrong direction!

Age

Like family history, age is, unfortunately, unmodifiable (not even with a little nip-and-tuck here and there). Part of the natural aging process is the development of heart disease, stroke, and cancer. These illnesses are associated with certain genes that are activated as we age. So we can say that the development of heart disease is genetically encoded and predetermined.

As we age, then, it becomes more important to screen for the early onset of certain conditions. Cholesterol can begin to harm the body at an early age. For this reason, a baseline total cholesterol level measurement is recommended at age 20. If that measurement is elevated, a measurement of the various cholesterol components (for instance, LDL, HDL, and triglyceride levels) is recommended. Based on those findings, a physician can begin recommending various lifestyle changes to lower those cholesterol levels. The goal here is to stop the damage (and reverse it) as soon as possible.

The Doctor Says

The natural aging process results in many diseases, such as cancer, heart disease, and stroke. By modifying certain lifestyle choices (such as diet and exercise), we can try to minimize the effects of aging.

We hope that one day age can become modifiable, but for now, the best we can do is to keep a close eye on the natural aging process and try to stop the negative effects in its tracks.

Gender

Sex is rapidly becoming less of a definitive risk factor. I'll discuss it here as a means of debunking the conventional wisdom that may still be circulating out there.

It was once believed that males were more prone to heart attacks and strokes than women, but now this belief is falling by the wayside. Doctors used to think that women were somewhat protected by female hormones against developing heart disease; however, heart disease is the leading killer of women in this country. And because physicians have determined that hormone replacement therapies are dangerous to women's health, we no longer believe that estrogen and progesterone offer any measure of protection against heart disease.

Before menopause, women develop heart disease about 10 years later than men do; after menopause, the rate of women's heart disease rapidly approaches that of their male counterparts. Moreover, heart disease in women is often more serious and likely to be fatal. Now, the difference in outcomes (survival versus death rates) may be attributed to how women with heart disease are diagnosed and treated (we're learning that women don't always present the classic signs of heart attack, for example), but a certain percentage is related to unknown factors.

Risk Factors You Can Change

Now for the good news: there are risk factors that you *do* have control over. You can modify these factors, and thereby reduce the risk of heart disease and stroke. Knowing that you *can* change certain risk factors is one thing; actually changing them and maintaining a healthy lifestyle requires dedication and vigilance.

The *cholesterol panel*, which consists of total cholesterol and its subfractions, is a powerful predictor of future health. The effects of lowering your cholesterol are multiplicative. The lower your total cholesterol, LDL, and triglycerides, the better your health will be. In other words, the main goal of modifying certain risk factors is to lower your cholesterol level. However, in doing this, you'll also improve your health, improve your quality of life, and increase your life span.

And there's even more you can do to your cholesterol levels to improve your health. Elevating your HDL levels provides even more protection against illness. This works even if you're not completely successful in lowering your total cholesterol, LDL, and triglyceride numbers. Raising HDL levels is a more difficult task than simply lowering total cholesterol. To review more about this topic, flip back to Chapter 3.

Let's take a look now at how you can target those modifiable risk factors and lower your cholesterol numbers.

Diet

A poor diet is a powerful risk factor for poor health. Heart attack, stroke, and cancers have all been linked to poor eating habits. Conversely, a healthy diet promotes good health.

The cells in our bodies renew themselves on a continuous basis, and they need healthy fuel to promote healthy regeneration. For example, when we're born, the lining of the inside of our blood vessels is so healthy that it can prevent a blood clot from forming on its surface by releasing various blood thinners. As we get older and eat high-fat foods, the cholesterol goes up (creating clogged arteries, blood clots, and the like) and our health goes down. We are truly what we eat, and all our cells need a healthy food supply to promote their continued good health.

Eating a healthy diet in the United States takes effort because so many of our food products are artificially processed to improve their taste. A diet rich in saturated fats drives up cholesterol levels and increases the likelihood of a person developing heart disease. On the other hand, a low-calorie diet that's also low in cholesterol and saturated fats will help to decrease cholesterol and improve that person's health.

So what should we be eating for optimum health? To lower cholesterol and minimize the chances for developing illnesses, we need to adopt the eating habits that nature intended for us. This means shifting our eating patterns to dramatically increase our intake of fruits, vegetables, and low-fat meats.

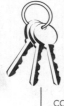

Here's to Your Heart

Primitive man ate what's known as a **Paleolithic diet,** which basically consisted of food that could be hunted or that came from the ground or the trees. In remote areas of the world, people still eat this way. Guess what? These people have low cholesterol levels; low blood pressure; and low incidences of diabetes, heart disease, and cancer. Mother Nature knows what's best for us!

In Chapter 7, we talk more about making more specific food choices in the interest of improving your health. But for now, let's consider a simple approach to changing the way we think about dieting. Being overweight is almost always a voluntary condition. That is, most of the time, excess weight is not caused by a medical condition, but by a person simply eating too many calories and not burning them off through some sort of physical activity. Those extra calories are stored as fat. Combine that stored fat with a sedentary lifestyle, and the result is elevated cholesterol levels and an increased risk for heart disease and stroke.

Here's to Your Heart

Consuming too many calories leads to weight gain and increased cholesterol levels. Elevated cholesterol and illness go hand-in-hand. By improving your diet and dropping to an ideal weight, you'll derive the added benefits of lower cholesterol and better health!

Because most foods (except "zero-calorie" foods) contain calories, we're all faced with deciding how many calories we're going to consume every day. Improving your health and lowering your cholesterol can be as easy as deciding what to eat and what not to eat. Now, if you aim for a diet consisting of low-calorie, nutritive foods, you don't have to diet in the traditional sense of the word.

Let's say you have a few extra pounds (and some extra cholesterol points) to shed. You can start improving your health by modifying your food choices. Perhaps in the morning, you can choose to use just one creamer in your coffee instead of two or three. Maybe after lunch, you'll choose to have an apple instead of a cupcake. And maybe at dinnertime, you'll pass up the gravy on your roasted turkey.

These are relatively small modifications, and they aren't a solution to long-term weight management—but they are a step in the right direction.

Exercise

Daily exercise helps lower cholesterol and improves health. It has also been shown to lower the risk of heart disease and stroke. A sedentary lifestyle (that is, the absence of physical activity) is a major risk factor in the development of poor health.

Over the years, researchers have been on a quest to determine how much exercise we need to remain healthy, and it turns out that we don't need all that much. We don't need to engage in strenuous activity or train to become professional athletes to reap the benefits of exercise; nor do we need to invest in a lot of expensive exercise equipment or spend money on a gym membership.

Everyone should shoot for about 30 minutes of moderate activity a day, which is doable for most people. And because these 30 minutes don't have to be consecutive (breaking them into 10-minute increments is just as good for your health), you can start by making some simple changes in your everyday behaviors. Walk to work instead of driving, if that's possible; and if it's not possible, take the farthest spot in the parking lot and squeeze some walking into your day that way.

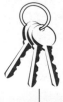

Here's to Your Heart

It's funny how people will drive around and around a parking lot, looking for a closer spot, or how they'll sit and wait for someone to leave a spot that's close to the entrance of a building. These people could already be in their office (or in the mall, or the grocery store) *and* have knocked out a few minutes worth of exercise if they had chosen the less desirable—but better-for-their-health—spot!

Another way to sneak some activity into your busy day is to take the stairs instead of the elevator. If you work on the twentieth floor and you know you'll just never make it all the way up that stairwell, then walk part of the way and take the elevator when you're out of steam. Or, if you have the time, walk part of the way, take a rest, and then continue up those steps.

Other ideas for increasing your daily activity level include using your bike instead of the car whenever possible, or taking the dog for a long walk each day. If you happen to live near a beach, a morning walk on the sand is an excellent form of exercise. Jump rope. Swim laps. Do some push-ups and sit-ups. Just find something you enjoy and get moving.

After exercise becomes part of your daily routine (like brushing your teeth), it becomes something you'll easily adhere to, and something you'll no longer dread—I promise. For more details on incorporating a fitness plan into your everyday life, turn to Chapter 15.

The Doctor Says

Medication is sometimes necessary for lowering cholesterol and should also be incorporated into a daily routine of heart-healthy activities (including healthy eating and exercise) when appropriate.

Multiple Risk Factors

Although targeting risk factors individually will lower your probability of developing heart disease and stroke, taking aim at several risk factors simultaneously will produce even better results. In fact, modifications that target one risk factor (like adjusting your diet) will naturally benefit other risk factors (like lowering your cholesterol).

def•i•ni•tion

Risk factor modification involves evaluating your various risk factors and changing them as needed to lower your chances of developing an illness.

Living a life of *risk factor modification* lowers cholesterol and keeps you healthy. To be successful in this goal, however, you must be conscientious in your daily routines and choices. If you can learn to include exercise and healthy foods into everyday life (targeting two risk factors simultaneously), you'll be able to lower your cholesterol (thereby minimizing a third risk factor!) and improve your health with less effort.

How Low Should You Go?

Recent studies have convinced us that previous cholesterol goals need to be reduced even farther. We're learning that there may not be a lower limit for cholesterol, and that we can theoretically shoot for the lowest levels we can achieve. Babies are born with total cholesterol levels of 40 and with LDL levels of 25. As we age, our cholesterol increases, but it stands to reason that the human body can tolerate low levels of cholesterol.

Doctors used to believe that cholesterol had to be reduced to a target number: the higher one's health risk, the lower the cholesterol needed to go. We also believed that once a person reached that goal, there was little benefit to further reducing cholesterol. However, we now know that if a person has multiple noncholesterol risk factors, his cholesterol level should be driven even lower than we previously thought.

Let's look at how specific recommendations for lowering cholesterol have recently changed:

> **Healthy Heart Facts**
>
> Non-cholesterol risk factors include smoking, obesity, advanced age, gender, a family history of heart disease or stroke, leading a sedentary lifestyle, and the presence of diabetes. When someone has multiple risk factors, any reduction in cholesterol, however small, will have beneficial effects.

- Doctors used to believe that if a person had diagnosed heart disease (a history of heart attack, for example), the LDL level should be less than 100 mg/dl.

- If a person had two or more risk factors for heart disease or stroke, the LDL level should be less than 130 mg/dl.

- If a person had only one risk factor, the LDL level should be less than 160 mg/dl.

The most up-to-date studies show that these levels should be reduced by 30 mg/dl! So as you can see, we're moving toward believing that where cholesterol is concerned, the lower, the better—and, regardless of the number of risk factors a person may have, there may be no such thing as too low.

Your Risk Factor Score

You can accurately assess your likelihood of developing heart disease or stroke by evaluating the combination of your risk factors. The *risk factor score* is determined by incorporating various risk factors into an integral score that predicts the probability of a person developing heart disease or stroke in the future. In other words, each risk factor is assigned a numerical value, and the final tally determines the likelihood of a person developing heart disease over time.

def•i•ni•tion

A **risk factor score** is a numerical assessment of a person's multiple risk factors for heart disease and stroke. One major consideration in this score is a person's cholesterol levels. The final score indicates the probability of heart disease or stroke in the future.

Physicians may use several different risk factor scores. The well-known and time-tested Framingham Score takes the following risk factors into consideration:

◆ Age

◆ Gender

◆ Total cholesterol level

◆ HDL level

◆ Diabetes

◆ History of smoking

◆ History of heart disease

A major element of this score (and, you'll note, the one modifiable factor listed here) is cholesterol and its components (namely, LDL, HDL, and triglycerides). Lowering your total cholesterol level (with the goal of reducing LDL and increasing HDL) decreases your risk factor score and, just as important, improves your overall health.

The Least You Need to Know

◆ Risk factors determine the likelihood of a person developing specific illnesses over time.

◆ Risk factors for heart disease and stroke include family history, age, poor diet, elevated cholesterol levels, and a sedentary lifestyle.

◆ Because some risk factors are impossible to change, we need to concentrate on those that we can modify, such as lowering cholesterol levels.

◆ Recent studies indicate that there may be no lower limit for reducing cholesterol.

◆ The Framingham Score is one tool doctors use to assess a person's risk factor score, which indicates the likelihood of heart disease or stroke in the future.

Chapter 6

Diagnosing Cholesterol Problems

In This Chapter

◆ Learn why you need to fast before a cholesterol screening.

◆ Understand why your doctor may order a series of tests along with your cholesterol panel.

◆ Read about the difference between angiogram and angioplasty.

◆ Discover the common procedures that are used to visualize the blood vessels and cholesterol buildup.

◆ Know the pros and cons of testing your cholesterol at home.

This book's purpose is to advise you on how to either prevent or correct elevated cholesterol. Obviously, if you don't know a problem exists, you can't work to improve the situation. Maybe you haven't yet been diagnosed with high cholesterol but have a family history of heart disease and are concerned, or perhaps, you've been told to lower your cholesterol levels but have no idea where your doctor is getting these seemingly random numbers from.

Whatever your situation—whether you know your specific cholesterol numbers or at this point are only concerned about where they may lie—this chapter fills you in on how doctors determine that a patient has high cholesterol and some of the tests they use to visualize the cardiovascular system.

Fast Results!

The simplest way to diagnose a cholesterol problem is to have a *fasting cholesterol panel* done. You'll remember from Chapter 1, a cholesterol panel is a blood test that breaks cholesterol down into its subfractions (HDL, LDL, and triglycerides). When cholesterol levels are broken down in this way, doctors have a much better idea of your level of health than they would have from looking at one total number for cholesterol. For example, high LDL levels combined with low HDL levels pose a much more significant risk to your health than an elevated HDL and low LDL.

def•i•ni•tion

A **fasting cholesterol panel** is a simple blood test obtained after a person has gone 8–12 hours without eating. It eliminates any error associated with raised triglyceride levels caused by eating, and it gives your doctor a clear idea of which cholesterol subfractions may be legitimately elevated.

Why Fast?

It's important for your cholesterol to be evaluated after a period of fasting because triglycerides levels can rise dramatically immediately after eating. Obviously, this can cause a spike that could be misinterpreted on your test results. But if you had a blood test done right after eating, a high triglyceride level is just as likely to be downplayed and attributed to the meal you've just consumed. If that triglyceride level is elevated in your bloodstream all the time, this is a threat to your health that you don't want overlooked!

In addition, triglyceride levels affect LDL levels. Although HDL and LDL levels change little after a person eats, LDL levels are calculated using a formula that incorporates triglycerides. So an elevated triglyceride level caused by a recent fatty meal can result in an inaccurate LDL reading, too.

Healthy Heart Facts

If your cholesterol panel comes back with elevated or abnormal levels of HDL, LDL, or triglycerides, your doctor will want to repeat the test to confirm the accuracy of the results.

For these reasons, it's simply in everyone's best interest to eliminate the possibilities for misinterpretation of test results. And because fasting isn't invasive and doesn't quite equate to physical torture, it's one of the easiest ways to ensure that cholesterol panel readings are accurate.

Reading Between the Lines

The various subfractions of a cholesterol panel should also be interpreted based on any underlying illness, such as thyroid disorders, liver problems, and diabetes. Various medications can also alter cholesterol subfraction values. For instance, various heart medications can affect LDL, HDL, and triglyceride levels. Most of these changes are minor; however, if there is any question about the accuracy of the results and whether underlying illnesses and disorders are playing a role in *creating* a cholesterol disorder, the panel should be repeated.

Medications usually cause only minimal fluctuations in the cholesterol components, so major cholesterol abnormalities are *unlikely* to be the result of medication.

While You've Got That Needle in Your Arm ...

Because you're fasting and having blood drawn *anyway*, a physician will often request that the lab perform additional tests. The tests that your doctor may ask for might be helpful in identifying other health risks and interpreting your cholesterol results in terms of your overall cardiovascular risk.

For example, along with the cholesterol panel, it's useful to obtain a *fasting glucose level*, which helps to determine whether a person is diabetic or prediabetic. A fasting blood sugar is highly useful because cholesterol disorders are much more dangerous in diabetics. Moreover, diabetes is highly underdiagnosed! It's estimated that *millions* of Americans have undiagnosed diabetes and have no idea that they are at risk for heart disease, amputations, and blindness! Millions more are prediabetic because of excess belly fat, poor diet, and lack of exercise.

def•i•ni•tion

A **fasting glucose level** measures the amount of sugar in the bloodstream and is often obtained along with a fasting cholesterol panel. Elevated glucose levels may mean that a person is diabetic or prediabetic. These conditions pose a threat to cardiovascular health, especially when combined with other risk factors (such as elevated cholesterol levels).

In addition, cholesterol disorders and diabetes typically occur together and increase risk *synergistically*. That means that these conditions don't just coexist in the body; they actually feed off of one another and make each condition worse than it would be on its own. (Kind of like how teenagers behave when they're in packs—individually, they may not be horrible, but put them together and watch out!)

The Doctor Says

Cholesterol disorders and elevated fasting blood sugar are both components of the metabolic syndrome (which were discussed in Chapter 4). Add the combination of these two factors to *other* risk factors—such as hypertension and obesity—and the risk for heart disease and stroke increases dramatically.

High Blood Pressure and Cholesterol Levels

Before you obtain a cholesterol profile, your physician is almost certain to measure your blood pressure and, if appropriate, discuss weight loss and smoking cessation. These risk factors are often seen in people with cholesterol disorders and significantly increase the risk of cardiovascular disease.

A systolic blood pressure in the 130s (which is below the 140 cutoff for high blood pressure) should be treated when other risk factors, such as diabetes and high cholesterol levels, exist. The treatment is often the same diet, exercise, and medications that are used to treat abnormal cholesterol. In fact, a recent landmark study showed that cholesterol-reducing medication helped control blood pressure in a group of people who had abnormal cholesterol levels.

The Doctor Says

Blood pressure is considered elevated with the systolic number hits 140. However, elevated blood pressure levels are usually minimal. Oftentimes, the systolic blood pressure will be 140 to 160, or even high normal (in the 130s). When other risk factors are involved, such as diabetes or raised levels of cholesterol, even marginally high blood pressure should be treated! Again, these conditions work together—against your health!

Lipoprotein Profile

We've actually been talking about lipoproteins throughout the course of this book. If you recall, HDL stands for high-density lipoprotein, and LDL (naturally) stands for low-density lipoprotein. But up to this point, we haven't actually defined lipoprotein. There's no time like the present…

Lipoproteins are combinations of lipid (fat) and protein. (Definitions just don't get much simpler than this.) All the cholesterol panel subfractions circulate in the blood as combinations of lipids and proteins. You'll recall from Chapter 1 that cholesterol is made up of protein. The central core of the cholesterol is formed by lipid, or fat. The proteins form the exterior of the cholesterol particle.

def•i•ni•tion

Cholesterol is composed of **lipoproteins,** which are compounds formed from lipid and protein. All the cholesterol subfractions are lipoproteins.

Lipoprotein Breakdown

Depending on the lab that you go to, your cholesterol panel will contain various measurements of the following, as well as various other cholesterol ratios:

- LDL
- HDL
- Triglycerides
- VLDL

"Now wait a minute," you're saying. "What's this *VLDL* all about?" VLDL stands for very low-density lipoprotein. VLDL is made by the liver and contains a very high proportion of triglycerides. Along with another subfraction called *IDL (intermediate density lipoprotein)*, VLDL increases the risk for heart disease.

The Doctor Says

In addition to HDL, LDL, and triglycerides, your doctor may also be interested in your **VLDL** (very low-density lipoprotein) and **IDL** (intermediate-density lipoprotein) levels, both of which increase the risk of heart disease in high levels. Any lipoprotein that is not HDL is referred to as **non-HDL cholesterol;** these values are of particular interest to a doctor who is evaluating your risk of cardiovascular disease.

We don't typically address these particular cholesterol subfractions individually. The therapies used for lowering LDL and triglycerides work for IDL and VLDL also.

IDL and VLDL are part of a new measurement called *non-HDL cholesterol*. Because the only good cholesterol is HDL, by subtracting HDL from total cholesterol, we're left with the bad subfractions: LDL, VLDL, IDL, and triglyceride. The goal is to get the non-HDL cholesterol down to less than 130 mg/dl.

Ratio Relevance

What doctors look for in a cholesterol panel—aside from the actual numbers—are the ratios of the numbers in relation to one another. The most common ratios we compare are HDL to LDL and vice versa. These ratios are a good indicator of how one's health is doing and where it's headed in the not-so-distant future.

Although the cutoff numbers for elevated risk vary from lab to lab, what we see too often is that as total cholesterol or LDL increases, HDL decreases. As a result, the ratio of LDL to HDL increases, and so does cardiovascular risk.

CRP

As with the fasting cholesterol panel, your doctor might also request the lab run some other important tests along with a lipoprotein profile to further assess your risk stratification (or where you lie in the greater picture of risk factors). One test he may request is called a *CRP (C-reactive protein)* measurement, which is a measure of inflammation in the body.

def•i•ni•tion

CRP (C-reactive protein) is made by the liver and reflects the overall level of inflammation in the body. Various stimuli, including infection, may increase CRP, and as the CRP increases, so does your risk for heart attack and stroke.

The combination of a high CRP, elevated LDL, and a low HDL is quite dangerous. In fact, the greater the number and degree of abnormalities in these test results, the higher the risk to your health is.

What's really interesting is that exercising and eating a healthy diet not only lower LDL and raise HDL, but also lower CRP, which in turn theoretically implies a decrease in the risk for heart attack and stroke. Now, the important word there is *implies*, because doctors have not yet proved that lowered CRP levels translate into fewer heart attacks and strokes—but it makes intuitive sense that this would be the case.

Healthy Heart Facts

Recent studies also support the theory that reducing CRP reduces cardiovascular risk. One baby aspirin (81 mg) helps reduce CRP. A group of male physicians were the subjects of a study where baby aspirin prevented first heart attacks. The aspirin prevented heart attacks only in those doctors who had elevated CRP at the beginning of the study. Of course, you shouldn't begin taking any medication without first consulting with your doctor.

Angiogram

No, it's not a test for a woman named Angie O. Gram, but a vital tool in your cardiologist's office that can be used to assess the state of your blood vessels. Although angiograms do give us a good idea of what's going on inside your arteries, they aren't perfect. For one thing, they're rather invasive (requiring a local anesthetic and an incision). In addition, doctors don't always get the full story on cholesterol build-up from this test.

The Story Leading Up to the Angiogram

Typically, individuals with elevated cholesterol and other risk factors for heart disease note a decrease in their ability to tolerate exercise, or they might have chest pains or shortness of breath with exertion. (They might be huffing and puffing after taking walks, for example.) What may be happening is that these individuals have a blockage in an artery that has become so advanced that blood isn't being supplied to the heart in sufficient amounts.

Whenever demand must go up, such as when a person exercises, supply must go up as well. If supply cannot go up because the artery is narrowed, there is a supply-demand mismatch, which the heart experiences as pain or discomfort.

This is a classic supply-and-demand mismatch problem, and it usually occurs in multiple blood vessels all over the body. Cholesterol deposition and inflammatory cell accumulation on the inside of the blood vessels cause narrowings, or *stenoses*, which can eventually block the flow of blood altogether. You'll remember, though, that back in Chapter 2 you read that your arteries can compensate for these

def•i•ni•tion

A **stenosis** is a narrowing of an artery. (Several narrowings are called **stenoses.**) The blood vessels will sometimes compensate for a stenosis by developing collaterals around the blockage or by actually increasing in diameter.

stenoses by forming collaterals or bypasses around the narrowed areas. Arteries also have an amazing ability to increase in diameter (what doctors call remodeling) to allow for increased blood flow. For these reasons, symptoms of the blockage typically aren't felt until the artery is 70–90 percent blocked! At this point, there's little the arteries can do to compensate for the damage that's been done. This is when people start to feel chest pains or—unfortunately—suffer heart attacks. Determining *which* artery will cause the heart attack is difficult.

The Doctor Says

Even with our advanced diagnostic tools, it's just not possible to say *which* artery will contribute to a heart attack. Consider this: Most heart attacks occur in an artery with 40% to 60% blockage, rather than in arteries with blockage of 90% or better. How could this be? An artery that is 90% occluded will develop collaterals, or little blood vessel sprouts, that bypass the blockage altogether, something that arteries with lesser blockage don't do. It's *more* likely that an artery with 90% blockage will become suddenly occluded; however, less severe blockages are more common. Statistically speaking, then, it's more likely for a heart attack to be the result of a lesser blockage.

What to Expect from an Angiogram

Angiogram is one technique that has been used to identify localized plaque rupture. This is an x-ray study that your cardiologist may perform to visualize the degree of blockage in your blood vessels. Here's what this test entails:

- The patient lies on a table.

- The cardiologist numbs the area around the femoral artery, which is a major artery located in the groin area.

- The cardiologist inserts a catheter into the lumen (opening) of the blood vessel.

- He threads the catheter up along the artery toward the heart.

- Using the guidance of the x-ray machine, the cardiologist inserts the catheter into the lumen of the arteries that supply blood to the heart.

- After the catheter is in place, the doctor then injects contrasting dye that will show up on an x-ray.

The purpose of the contrast is to show the degree to which a blood vessel has become narrowed. So when all is said and done, the angiogram gives the doctor a good idea of what kind of blockages you may be dealing with.

Angioplasty

Obviously, the benefit of knowing that a particular blood vessel is in bad shape is that we can attempt to correct the situation. Maybe you know of someone who went in for an angiogram and came out scheduled for angioplasty. So, you wonder, what went on there?

Based upon the degree of narrowing of the blood vessels, cardiologists may recommend a balloon procedure, or *angioplasty*, to open the narrowed blood vessel. The balloon is inserted in much the same way that angioplasty is performed, except that when the catheter reaches the area of blockage, the balloon is actually inflated within the artery, which pushes the mushy cholesterol out of the way, like a snow plow. When the cholesterol is moved out of the way of the flowing blood, this typically relieves the symptoms of chest pain upon exertion.

Often a *stent* is placed to hold the vessel open. This device looks like a piece of chicken wire and allows the blood vessel to remain open, as many blood vessels—as many as one third to one half—will renarrow after angioplasty.

def•i•ni•tion

Angioplasty is sometimes performed to open a narrowed artery. In this procedure, a balloon is opened inside the artery and moves the cholesterol or plaque out of the opening of the blood vessel. A **stent,** something that looks like chicken wire, may be placed in the blood vessel during angioplasty to prevent renarrowing.

The Doctor Says

When multiple arteries are critically narrowed, a bypass operation may be required. Bypass surgery utilizes arteries and veins from other areas the body to reroute the blood flow around the narrowings. Bypass surgery is similar to detouring traffic around closed lanes on a freeway or highway. Double bypass surgery implies that two arteries need re-routing; triple bypass implies that there are three arteries involved, and so on.

The Limitations of Angiograms

When critical narrowings or stenoses aren't seen on an angiogram, you won't need bypass surgery or angioplasty, which you might take to be the best possible news. But as long as your cholesterol numbers remain elevated, medical therapy, including diet, exercise, and medications will still be needed. In fact, these therapies will be needed *even if* the patient *also* needs angioplasty or bypass surgery.

Procedures such as angioplasty and bypass surgery do not prevent heart attacks. *Cholesterol reduction and risk factor modification prevent heart attacks!* Although there may be no role for angioplasty, stenting, or bypass surgery for moderate blockages, the danger of *intermediate stenoses* (blockages that are not as severe in degree as the major narrowings but are just as potentially life threatening) is that most heart attacks occur in these areas, and yet, they often don't show up on angiography!

A blood vessel may be up to 40 percent narrowed and still appear healthy on angiography. This is due to the remodeling process that we discussed earlier; the blood vessels can actually grow in diameter to accommodate for the plaque on the blood vessel wall. Because the angiogram really only visualizes the lumen of the blood vessel and not the wall (you could say the angiogram is really only a "lumenogram"), someone could have an angiogram showing wide open blood vessels and still suffer a heart attack.

Ultrasound

Ultrasound technology was originally developed in the 1940s in the form of sonar. The military used sonar to detect submarines and to map the bottom of the ocean. This same technology can map the structure of the heart. Although people usually think of expectant mothers when they hear *ultrasound* this test has been used for several decades to diagnose heart disease.

The Basics of Ultrasound

Ultrasound is a type of sound wave that has a high frequency. Humans hear sound within a narrow frequency range. Dogs, on the other hand, hear sound of a higher frequency. Ultrasound is of an even higher frequency and is out the range of a dog's hearing.

Ultrasound works by producing pictures with sound waves. A crystal is stimulated with electricity, which causes the crystal to vibrate extremely rapidly. These vibrations produce a sound wave (ultrasound), which can be focused in the form of a beam. This beam can penetrate the chest wall and be used to create an image of the heart.

The ultrasound image is created by a computer that measures the time it takes for the reflected ultrasound waves to return to the crystal. The farther away from the crystal a structure is within the heart, the longer it takes for the sound waves to return and be detected by the computer. The computer integrates the information from millions of sound wave beams to create an image in real time of the heart beating. Check out the illustration of sound waves for a clearer picture of how this technology works.

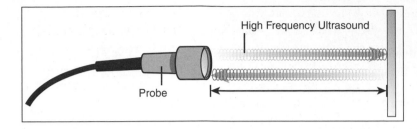

High Frequency Ultrasound

Probe

As ultrasound waves bounce off of a target, we can determine the distance between the source of the sound waves and the target (in this case, the heart). From these measurements, ultrasound helps us to visualize the image itself.

Advances in Ultrasound

The device that contains the crystal and creates the ultrasound beam is called a *transducer*. Recently, teeny transducers were created that can be passed along a wire down a blood vessel under x-ray guidance. The device sits atop the wire much like a monorail (which, is, in fact the name given to the system that passes the transducer down the lumen of the blood vessel).

Why is this important? This transducer can create an image of the cholesterol within blood vessels! By studying these images, doctors have learned that blood vessels that appear wide open on angiograms may actually harbor significant atherosclerosis. Even more remarkably, medications that reduce cholesterol have been shown to reduce the amount of atherosclerosis on the inside of blood vessels. How do we know this? The regression of plaque has been measured using ultrasound. In addition, ultrasound has been used to help determine which areas within the blood vessels harbor cholesterol deposits that are prone to rupture and lead to heart attacks.

Sounds great, right? So why aren't we using this technique on every patient, all the time? The difficulty with applying this technology is that it's invasive. A person typically has to undergo an angiogram to benefit from this technology. In addition, imaging the coronary arteries requires x-ray radiation. Therefore, a puncture and x-ray exposure are required to deploy a transducer down an artery to visualize the cholesterol within the wall of the blood vessel.

Healthy Heart Facts

There remains a need to create a technology that can image cholesterol deposits within a blood vessel without entering the body. CT scans and MRIs are two such potential technologies, but there are many other complex technologies on the horizon that will potentially evaluate the amount of cholesterol within the wall of a blood vessel. Even more important is the potential ability to determine which area of the blood vessel wall is prone to rupture and may lead to a heart attack. Application of this technology may be able to prevent heart attacks in the future.

CT Scans

Recently, coronary calcium scanning tests have become available. *Coronary CT (computerized tomography)* is a technique wherein the amount of calcium within the coronary arteries is quantified.

def•i•ni•tion

Calcification is a process wherein calcium crystals are deposited within the blood vessels. If cholesterol sits for a long enough period of time, it can calcify in the arteries. This process is thought to actually make the cholesterol plaque more stable and less likely to rupture.

Coronary CT (computerized tomography) is a diagnostic test used to assess the amount of calcium within the coronary arteries.

We know that the soft cholesterol that deposits on the inside of the arteries is especially dangerous because it's prone to rupture and cause a heart attack. Cholesterol deposits that have been in the blood vessels for a long time can *calcify*. Theoretically, longstanding atherosclerotic plaque is relatively stable, especially if it has calcified, because this hardening may decrease the likelihood of rupture. However, this is only a theory, and we know that plaque rupture can and does occur in calcified areas.

Think of this as a plumbing problem. The more debris deposited on the inside of the pipes (or, actually, blood vessels), the greater the burden of the debris. Plaque burden correlates with increased risk. The more plaque building up, the greater the risk of some of it rupturing. Although some plaque will calcify and that this may stabilize the plaque, doctors worry about the amount of plaque. If you have a little bit of plaque, there will be a little bit of calcium. But if your coronary scan shows a lot of calcium, it means you have a lot of plaque (and also suggests you have advanced cardiovascular disease). The more plaque, the greater the heart-attack risk, whether it has calcified or not.

Although CT scans are popular, because risk factors for heart disease can be easily determined in any given patient, an expensive CT scanner with radiation exposure seems rather unnecessary. Plus, we don't glean rock-solid information from coronary CT scans: a positive scan does not necessarily mean that someone will have a heart attack, and a negative scan does not necessarily imply lack of atherosclerotic heart disease.

Home Cholesterol Tests

Home cholesterol tests have been on the market for a number of years. You can find them in most pharmacies and they're relatively inexpensive, and although these tests vary, most are up to 95 percent accurate. Some of the cholesterol tests only indicate total cholesterol, whereas others provide a subfraction analysis (breaking that total number down into HDL, LDL, triglycerides, and so on).

The major problem with home cholesterol testing is that most people aren't able to take the number from the test and integrate it into an overall cardiovascular assessment of risk without the help of a physician. The results of a home cholesterol test might easily allow you to diagnose a cholesterol disorder, but unless you have some training in the field of cardiovascular medicine, it's *not* easy to look at those results and say, "Ah ha! I know *exactly* what I need to do to eliminate all of my other risk factors and lead a healthier life!" That's where your cardiologist can be of significant assistance.

In addition, because the guidelines in recent years have recommended lower LDL levels, it's possible to under diagnose the seriousness and severity of your cholesterol abnormalities and assume that your risk is lower than it actually is. Also, although your total cholesterol may be normal, the subfractions may be dramatically *abnormal* and increase risk substantially.

For example, mildly elevated LDL and triglyceride levels combined with a low HDL increase your risk substantially, because the ratio of LDL or total cholesterol to HDL may be more important than your overall cholesterol number. Although home tests can give you an idea of where your cholesterol levels are, to fully appreciate the severity of lipid disorders and the risk that they pose to your health, you need to have your test results evaluated by a physician with expertise in cardiovascular diseases.

> **Healthy Heart Facts**
>
> The world of medicine is becoming increasingly specialized. Cholesterol disorders are being increasingly treated by doctors with special expertise in lipid management, called *lipidologists*.

The Least You Need to Know

- For the most accurate results, it's necessary to fast 8–12 hours before a cholesterol panel is performed.

- Testing for other disorders, such as diabetes, along with a cholesterol screening helps a doctor to gain a clearer understanding of a person's overall health risks.

- Angiogram involves the usage of a catheter inserted into the blood vessel, the injection of contrast dye, and an x-ray.

- ◆ Angioplasty is a procedure that involves opening a balloon in a narrowed artery to clear debris.

- ◆ Home cholesterol tests may be accurate in their numbers, but lack the follow-up that a doctor will provide.

Part 2

Nutrition for Lower Cholesterol

Do you desire your doughnuts? Love your lemon meringue? Can't sleep without your sweets? In Part 1, you learned about some of the ways in which cholesterol becomes elevated in the body, and I mentioned that food—specifically fat-laden food—is often one of the biggest culprits.

There's good news and there's bad news. The bad news first: scientists have not yet found a healthy way to produce doughnuts. But the good news is that there are many, many ways to modify your diet and make it heart-healthy! And "healthy" does *not* have to mean boring! The chapters in Part 2, teach you how to eat (and drink) as though your life depends on it … because it just might.

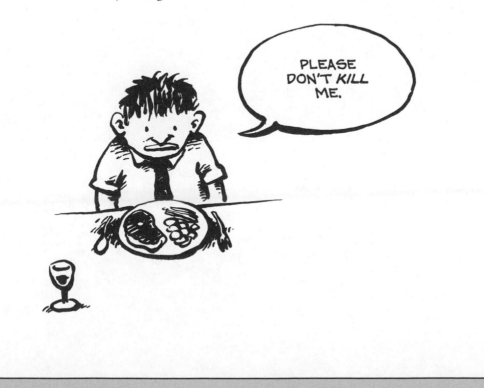

7

Heart-Smart Eating

In This Chapter

- ◆ Understand what calories do for the body and how they're stored
- ◆ Compare today's inactive, fat-consuming lifestyles with the way people used to live
- ◆ Get a sample of the best heart-healthy diets
- ◆ Take a virtual shopping trip for healthy foods

From the time we're born until the day we die, the way we eat has a powerful influence on our health. The result of extended life spans in developed nations, such as the United States and the countries in Western Europe, Australia, and New Zealand, is an epidemic of heart disease. The reason for this is simple. By the time humans reach old age, as they're more likely to do if they reside in developed nations (where food and healthcare are not the luxuries that they are in third-world countries), they have been exposed to decades of excess calories, high-fat diets, lack of exercise and a sedentary lifestyle. So for all the medical advances that allow us to live longer, we're still hurting ourselves by scarfing down too much fat and not working enough activity into our lives!

To decrease cholesterol and the risk for dangerous diseases (such as heart disease and diabetes), we have to shift our eating habits. While it would be ideal for this to begin at the societal level (where everyone would embrace fresh produce and shun drive-through food), people have to be responsible for the food that goes into their bodies. And although adopting healthy eating habits *should* begin in childhood, it's *never* too late to modify one's diet to reduce cholesterol and the risk for illness!

Nutrition Basics

Modifying your diet to achieve lower cholesterol and reduce the risk for heart disease is a relatively simple task. Making the right food choices isn't difficult in the short term (when you're excited about changing your lifestyle and improving your health),

Here's to Your Heart

Parents should do their best to instill healthy eating values in their children. If they're a regular part of a child's life, kids are more likely to stick with healthy eating habits as they age. Of course, parents should adhere to the same healthy eating habits and food choices that they make for their children.

but can be more difficult to adhere to over the long haul. The key to maintenance of healthy dietary habits is to keep yourself vigilant and motivated. Eating properly requires effort on a regular basis.

Unfortunately, most people who change their diets for the sake of improving their health eventually relapse into their old eating patterns. The new, healthier food choices become replaced with older, high-fat, high-cholesterol choices as time passes. There are powerful stimuli in our everyday environments that lure us into substituting healthy food with less healthy food, especially when unhealthy food rewards the eater with greater immediate pleasure.

Certainly, high-fat and high-calorie foods are tasty and enjoyable to eat. Generally, raw vegetables are less tasty than cheeseburgers are—for most of us, anyway—and it can take as much willpower to consume healthy foods as it does to turn away from unhealthy choices.

Effort is another issue when it comes to eating healthy foods. Surely, it's easier to open a bag of chips than to prepare a salad for a snack. However, the added effort of preparing healthy foods is well worth the health benefits. Some people also complain that healthy eating is too expensive. Here's where even more effort comes into play: Watch for sales at the supermarket. Buy vegetables in their most natural state — not pre-washed and pre-cut, niceties which tend to add to their prices.

Just the (Food) Facts

The basic concepts of healthy eating are simple. Here they are, summed up in two little, easy-to-recall points: (1) keep your daily *caloric* intake low, and (2) eat plenty of fruits, vegetables, and natural foods. (You know you're not getting off that easy, though. The reasoning behind these points follows.)

When we take in more calories than we use, the excess calories are stored as fat for future use. This is really an adaptive mechanism of the body that dates back to prehistoric times, when storage of energy was an insurance policy against future periods of food scarcity. Now, this adaptive mechanism was helpful when humans were hunters and gatherers. Thousands of years ago, humans lived from meal to meal; if food wasn't available, people didn't eat.

def•i•ni•tion _____

A **calorie** is a measure of how much potential energy is in a particular food. The definition of a calorie for biological systems is the amount of energy necessary to raise 1,000 grams of water by 1 degree Centigrade. Using this definition, all foods can be compared to one another based upon how much energy is stored within the food.

Obviously, this is not the case in our highly industrialized modern societies where we're bombarded with advertisements for food all the time! In fact, we don't even have to go out to look for food (not that visiting the grocery store is exactly comparable to the days of hunting and gathering). We can make a phone call and have our food delivered without ever having to leave that comfy seat in front of the TV (except to pay the delivery guy, of course)!

When we consume more food than we need for our immediate energy usage, some of that energy is stored within muscles (as a complex sugar called glycogen) and some is stored in the organs and under the skin—as fat. And that's the fat of the story.

How and Why Food Ends Up as Fat

When foods are consumed, they are digested by enzymes in the stomach and intestines. These enzymes break the complex food molecules down into simpler molecules, which are then transported by the blood to all of the cells in the body. The cells use these simpler molecules to provide energy for their own processes. They utilize other enzymes to break these simpler molecules down into even smaller molecules.

Ultimately, the energy that held the complex molecules together is captured and used by all the cells in the body to perform their basic functions. Whatever is left over is stored.

Calories In = Calories Out

There are really two ways to lose fat or decrease the amount of energy that is stored as fat. The first is to eat fewer calories. Simply put, calories in must equal calories out.

The best way to eat fewer calories is to eat foods that are lower in calories. For example, fat is a highly efficient way to store calories. The *purpose* of fat is to store calories, and pound for pound, more energy can be stored in fat than in muscle or in other bodily functions and systems. As a result, foods that have a high fat content have high caloric (energy) content.

Because a small amount of fat has so much energy, eating a high-fat meal can provide thousands of calories in one sitting, which is far more calories than are needed for basic cell functions. In addition, the fat is dangerous to the blood vessels. So not only does high-fat food provide excess calories that are ultimately stored as fat, it also damages blood vessels after consumption and for a long time afterward by elevating cholesterol.

Good Versus Bad Fats

As we discussed in Chapter 4, fats are composed of long chains of carbon atoms of variable lengths, surrounded by hydrogen atoms and attached to an alcohol backbone called glycerol. The more hydrogen atoms surrounding the carbon atoms, the more saturated the molecules are. The more saturated the fat, the more detrimental to our health. Consuming few saturated fats is healthiest for one's diet.

The Doctor Says

Examples of bad fats are palm oil, palm kernel oil, and coconut oils. These tropical oils raise LDLs and increase the risk for heart disease. Examples of foods that contain unhealthy or saturated fats are fried foods; lard; fatty meats, including lamb, bacon, and sausage; butter; and other dairy products. Healthier fats include safflower, sunflower, corn, canola, cottonseed, peanut, and olive oils.

Why We Need Fat

Earlier in this chapter, we discussed how fats are necessary components of our bodies. Our cells need fats to perform their basic functions. The nervous systems, for example, use fats as essential components of the layer of material that covers nerves and allows for nerve conduction. In addition, certain essential vitamins—specifically, A, D, E, and K—can only be absorbed with fat's assistance. The key to fat consumption is to consume foods that contain healthy fats as opposed to unhealthy fats.

Certain fats are necessary for life; these are called *essential fatty acids*. Two of these fatty acids are *linoleic* acid and *linolenic* acid. Linoleic acid is called an omega-6 fatty acid. This tells us that there is a double bond between two carbons and, as a result, less hydrogen. Another type of fatty acid, called omega-3 fatty acid, of which linolenic acid is an example, is found in fish oils. These fatty acids have a powerful effect on the cell membranes, or the fatty coat that surrounds every cell in the body. We'll talk more about the omega-3 fatty acids in the next section.

def•i•ni•tion

Essential fatty acids are fatty compounds that are necessary for basic cell functions.

Omega-3: The Fish Oil

Omega-3 fatty acids are anticlotting and anti-inflammatory. They reduce risk of heart attack and stroke.

When someone eats omega-3 fatty acids, the membranes of the cells that are responsible for blood inflammation, blood clotting, and heart attacks become filled with omega-3 fatty acids. When omega-3 fatty acids replace other fatty acids in the membranes surrounding the cells that are responsible for deadly heart attacks, the cells become less likely to form blood clots. Fish is an excellent source of omega-3 fatty acids.

Paleolithic Diet

Over millions of years of evolution, our bodies (and the bodies of other animals in the animal kingdom) have become dependent upon consuming certain dietary components that are necessary for optimum health. Eating a diet rich in foods that are easily obtained from the environment is associated with low incidence of heart disease, diabetes, cancer, and other ailments. The ideal diet for optimum health (and the one I recommend to my own patients) is the Paleolithic diet, which includes only foods that can be found in nature. The Paleolithic diet has fostered humans for thousands of years. You can't find this diet in a book; it's more of a mindset, a way of thinking about the food that goes into your body and what it does once you consume it. Does the food *you* eat build your body up and clean your body out, or does it simply clog up the works? The Paleolithic diet is a means of making the body healthier and stronger.

Change Is Not Always Good

Over the last two centuries or so, the lifestyles of Americans and people living in the industrialized nations of Western Europe have changed dramatically. Our lifestyles nowadays are a far cry from those of our prehistoric ancestors. Consider the following:

♦ **There has been an increase in caloric consumption.** With the affluence of modern society has come an increase in caloric consumption. Increased food consumption has facilitated the current epidemic of obesity and related diseases.

♦ **The foods we eat are high in fat.** Healthy, natural foods that contain healthy fats and low or moderate caloric content have been replaced with foods that are high in unhealthy saturated fats, cholesterol, and excess calories.

♦ **There has been a decrease in exercise.** The primary cause of the sedentary lifestyle is the invention of the automobile and a shift from work- and leisure-related *physical* activity to nonphysical activity. For example, consider how much time the average person spends commuting to work by car only to spend the day at a desk.

The combination of these three forces has laid the groundwork for the modern epidemics of heart disease, diabetes, obesity, and other illnesses.

This Change Is for the Best!

The Paleolithic diet does not include foods that are common in many people's everyday repertoire. Here are some samples of foods that are created by modern technologies and are laden with calories. These food choices were not available to human who lived thousands of years ago:

♦ Soft drinks and beverages containing high-fructose corn syrup and refined sugar

♦ Pastries and baked goods including cookies and cakes

♦ All candies and sweets

♦ Fried foods of all kinds

♦ Butter, margarine, mayonnaise, and foods containing lard

♦ Refined flour and sugar

You'd be hard pressed to find anthropological evidence of cavemen drinking soda and snacking on candy bars. You'd also be hard-pressed to find anthropological evidence of rampant heart disease, diabetes, and obesity dating back to the Paleolithic age.

The dietary choices of humans who lived thousands of years ago comprised a Paleolithic diet. By attempting to model the eating habits of humans who lived before the development of modern technologies, we can decrease cholesterol and the risk for heart disease. Adapting to the Paleolithic diet consists of substituting modern food choices (such as those on the previous list) with the following:

- Fruits
- Vegetables
- Fish
- Lean meats
- Poultry
- Legumes
- Beans
- Nuts
- Grains and cereals

Essentially, any food item that grows on a tree, sprouts from the ground, or is obtained by hunting is on the Paleolithic menu. You won't have to go to the extremes of growing, picking, or killing your own food to eat more healthfully—but if you're into that kind of thing, go for it!

The Doctor Says

What about the South Beach Diet, Atkins, or the other diets that are so popular right now? As a group, medical doctors don't endorse these diets for a simple reason: Our bodies *need* certain foods, like those included in the Paleolithic diet. The human body has functioned for thousands of years by utilizing nutrients found in nature. The answer to healthy eating, then, is not to deprive ourselves of carbohydrates or meat—the answer is to do away with *processed* foods and get back to the way we were meant to eat!

Mediterranean Diet

Picture yourself lounging on the shores of the Mediterranean. When it's time to drag yourself off the beach for lunch, are you going to order a burger and fries? Not if you look at the people around you, who will appear to be a healthy lot, thanks to the foods they use regularly in their diets.

The Mediterranean diet is low in refined flour, sugar, and saturated fat and has been associated with a reduced incidence of heart disease. Substitution of saturated fats with olive oil leads to a decrease in the risk for heart disease. Although this diet leaves saturated fat behind, it's rich in fruits, vegetables, whole grain cereals, legumes, chicken, and fish.

You can easily implement elements of the Mediterranean diet into your own kitchen on a daily basis. In addition to preparing meals containing the main elements of this diet, you can use olive oil instead of vegetable oil or butter when cooking. You can also ask for your food to be cooked in olive oil instead of butter or margarine when you're eating out.

The Doctor Says

Although specialized types of olive oil (extra virgin, cold-pressed, etc) are very low in fat, they also tend to be very expensive. It's really not necessary to go to these lengths to derive health benefits from olive oil. Most of the benefits come from simply making the switch from saturated fats (like butter) to unsaturated fats (like olive oil). Take the money you might have spent on extra-virgin olive oil and put it towards fruits and veggies!

DASH Diet

DASH (Dietary Approaches to Stop Hypertension) is an acronym for a study conducted that was initially conducted to evaluate the role of diet in controlling hypertension (high blood pressure). The study proved that a healthy diet lowers blood pressure. In the study, people with heart disease were given a healthy diet consisting of fruits and vegetables. They were then compared with another group who were given a placebo diet. The first group showed a reduction in heart disease–related events, such as heart attack and stroke.

The Mediterranean diet and DASH diets are heart-healthy diets. They control cholesterol and are close in nature to the Paleolithic diet.

The Paleolithic diet is, theoretically, the ideal diet because it uses food sources and nutrients present in the environment thousands of years before modern technological processing techniques. We just need to get back to basics and give our bodies the types of foods that they need and can easily use—*without* resorting to storing excess fat.

The Mediterranean diet and DASH diets control cholesterol and are heart-healthy diets. If you take a close look at the elements of each diet, you'll notice that they're very close in nature to the Paleolithic diet. Any one of these diets is a healthy means of taking control of your health; personally, I recommend the Paleolithic diet to my patients, as I feel it's the most beneficial to the cardiovascular system. In the following section, we'll talk about how to stock your home with healthy staples.

> **Healthy Heart Facts**
>
> The DASH diet consists of fruits, vegetables, legumes, nuts, seeds, and low-salt foods. It's closely related to the Paleolithic diet.

Sample Menus

Creating a healthy menu starts with the trip to the supermarket, which will be comparable to the hunt for meat or the gathering of plant foods that humans who lived thousands of years ago engaged in. View the trip to the market as a quest to obtain the foods that are on the Paleolithic menu. (But leave your spear at home. The prison system in this country doesn't offer the Paleolithic diet.)

Gathering in the Grocery Store

To obtain a cart filled with Paleolithic foods, view your refrigerator as a part of your stomach outside of your body, because anything you put into the refrigerator is likely to end up in your stomach. As you stock your refrigerator, ask yourself whether this item is part of the Paleolithic diet and whether it's healthy. Each and every food item should be examined with these questions in mind.

Most foods in the market are relatively easy to discern as healthy or unhealthy. *Healthy* and *unhealthy* should be the only two distinctions you make between foods. (*Not* sweet or salty, *not* chocolate or nonchocolate. *Healthy* or *unhealthy*.) Only healthy food should make it back to your refrigerator and into your body.

The Picky Paleolithic Shopper

It's important to realize that most of the foods in a supermarket are not part of the Paleolithic diet. In other words, it will be somewhat difficult, although not impossible, to find foods in the supermarket that should be a part of your Paleolithic diet, especially if you're not used to shopping for the freshest, from-the-earth foods. It's easy to prove

Here's to Your Heart _____

When you're looking for fresh foods in the grocery store, try to stay in the perimeter of the aisles. The produce, meat, fish, and dairy departments are typically located outside of those long aisles that contain the worst types of food.

to yourself that most foods in the market are *not* part of the Paleolithic diet. By simply reviewing the contents of each supermarket aisle, you can see that most of these foods are not fresh, they cannot be found in nature, and they should stay right where they are—on the shelves, gathering dust.

To start and maintain the Paleolithic diet, the most important component is to *purchase only* foods that are on the Paleolithic menu. Anything else that comes into the house *is* going to be eaten.

The Least You Need to Know

- ◆ Some fat is required by the body for basic cell functions.

- ◆ Calories not used for energy are stored as fat in the body.

- ◆ Modern technological advances have steered us away from eating the foods our bodies need and can use most efficiently.

- ◆ The ideal diet for humans is a Paleolithic diet.

8

Cholesterol-Lowering Foods

In This Chapter

◆ Read about the benefits of soy

◆ Dispel some of the myths that surround nuts

◆ Understand the disadvantages of eating refined grains

◆ Know why nutritional supplements can't hold a candle to consuming the real deal

◆ Understand how to substitute good fats for bad fats in your diet

Cholesterol-lowering foods consist of low-fat foods, such as fruits, vegetables, low-fat dairy products, nuts, legumes, grains, poultry, fish, and lean meat (basically, the elements contained in the Paleolithic diet, which we discussed in Chapter 7). These foods are chock-full of the nutrients that are necessary for our bodies' day-to-day functioning; in addition, as the name of this chapter suggests, they work with our bodies to clean out the gunk that accumulates inside of the blood vessel walls.

This chapter gives you a good overview of some of the healthiest foods available, along with an explanation of what makes each of these foods so good for you!

Soy Protein

Soy protein (which, as its name suggests, is derived from soybeans) has been shown to lower cholesterol. Good sources of soy include: tofu, soybeans, soynuts, soymilk, and soy yogurt.

In addition to packing a powerful protein punch, soy also contains protective substances called *phytoestrogens*. Phytoestrogens promote blood vessel health by allowing blood vessels to dilate efficiently when the need arises in tissues that they supply blood to. They act on the endothelium that lines the inside of blood vessels and, as a result, are anti-atherosclerotic.

def•i•ni•tion

Soy contains protective substances called **phytoestrogens**, which promote dilation of blood vessels and protect against heart disease and certain cancers. **Isoflavones** are one type of phytoestrogens.

One type of phytoestrogens is known as *isoflavones*. Isoflavones are antioxidants. These compounds prevent heart disease and cancer and can be found in many foods, including grapes and citrus fruits. It has been hypothesized that part of the protective effect of red wine against heart disease is through isoflavones.

Soy Many Antioxidants!

The quest for antioxidants has led the health-food industry to come up with tablets containing various vitamins, minerals, and other compounds with purported antioxidant properties. When taken by themselves, none of the vitamins or antioxidants has been shown to yield significant beneficial effects. However, eating foods rich in vitamins and antioxidants, such as soy, has been shown to have a positive effect on health. So here's a perfect example of how eating as nature intended us to eat (which, by the way, does *not* include ingesting nutrients in tablet form) can improve our health.

The idea that nutrients should be obtained through foods (as opposed to pills) is nothing new. There is really no escape from or a healthier substitute for eating a healthy diet. But *why* can't pills give us what we need? It's likely that foods contain many healthy substances, many of which remain undiscovered, that have to be consumed together (and in the form of natural food products) to give us the most beneficial effects. The best way to obtain the benefits of individual nutrients is to follow the Paleolithic diet. (For more info on this diet, read Chapter 7.)

Healthy Heart Facts

The evolution of plants and animals over millions of years has led to plants producing compounds that regulate the biochemistry of animals. For example, phytoestrogens closely resemble the human hormone estrogen. There are many substances that plants produce to regulate human metabolism. Many manmade drugs and pharmaceuticals are derived from plants. This interrelationship between plants and animals further proves that the Paleolithic diet is ideal. Although nature continues to give our bodies the best it has to offer, the modern-day departure from natural eating habits has led to the rise of heart disease and cancer (in addition to rising cholesterol levels and diabetes).

Nuts!

Nuts are just tree seeds that are covered by a shell. They're an excellent source of protein and vitamins. Contrary to what you may have heard in the past, nuts are healthy. Nuts contain many healthy compounds that protect against disease; however (believe it or not), most of these compounds are unknown, even in this day and age of modern science and technological advances! (Those nuts just continue to elude us!)

We do know that one of the fatty acids in nuts is called linolenic acid, which falls into the category of omega-3 fatty acids (the same type of fatty acids that are found in fish). Omega-3 fatty acids not only help reduce LDL and raise HDL, but they are also anti-inflammatory and anticlotting.

Walnuts are an excellent source of omega-3 fatty acids. A Harvard study looked at the combination of walnuts as a supplement to a Mediterranean diet and found that walnuts reduced total cholesterol and LDL. Different nuts have different levels of saturated and unsaturated fatty acids. Those with unsaturated fatty acids are preferable.

Healthy Heart Facts

Linolenic acid is an essential omega-3 fatty acid. Omega-3 fatty acids are heart healthy and may have anticancer effects. Linolenic acid can be obtained from nuts and flaxseed oil.

Nuts are high in fat, and therefore, should be used moderately. For example, coconut and palm kernel oils are highly saturated and should be avoided. The nuts with the highest fat and saturated fat content are macadamia nuts, Brazil nuts, and cashews. So go ahead and eat those nuts—but remember: everything in moderation.

Oats and Barley

Oats and barley belong to a class of foods called grains, which are the seeds of grasses. Grasses, meanwhile, are components of the Paleolithic diet, and you know by now that the Paleolithic diet is ideal for heart health!

One of the biggest differences between the way we eat today and the way humans ate centuries ago is that our wheat products are often refined—that is, the natural grains are actually removed from the food before we eat it. Because many nutrients are contained in those grains, we end up missing out on some essential vitamins and minerals.

Refined Is Not So Fine

For thousands of years, people ate grains in their natural form. People went out and picked the wheat, smashed it up, and made their breads. There were no factories spitting out presliced loaves. And *white* bread? There was no such thing!

During the last century, the refining process, which converts grains into breads, began to modify those grains. Although grains contain necessary and nutritious ingredients, such as essential fats, B vitamins, and fiber, the refining process removes these components and adds simple sugars and nonessential and dangerous fats. For example, the refining process converts wheat to pies, cakes, rolls, and pastries. These foods are not nutritious and have dangerous fats.

You can say—honestly—that refining grains takes out everything that nature intended us to ingest and adds substances that aren't good for us. Compare the nutrition label on a package of white bread to the label on a package of whole-grain bread. Then read the ingredients. You'll be *amazed* at the difference in the amount of nutrition, and disturbed by what you're ingesting along with that white bread. (Bleach, for example, is in that bread. And just as an aside, bleach is *not* on the list of heart-healthy foods.)

It's Raining Grain!

You don't have to look hard to find whole grains. Common examples include these foods, corn, rice, oats, millet, rye, barley, and wheat.

These grains contain a seed, called a *germ*, and a covering, called a *hull* or *bran*. The covering contains the nutrients. There is also a food component for the seed called *endosperm*. The refining process *removes* the bran and its nutrients and fatty acids. Ezekial Bread and breads bought in health food stores have a reliable grain content. When browsing the bread aisle in the supermarket, read the labels very carefully— look for breads that are made from whole grain and do *not* contain bleached white flour.

The Doctor Says

All grains, including oats and barley, should be consumed in their natural forms. You can find natural grains in granolas, natural cereals, and in their most natural states in health-food stores. And don't think that you have to sit down with a bowl of dry grain and force yourself to eat it. Sprinkle your grains over salads or add them to soups. They add an interesting crunch to your meals!

Flaxseed

Flaxseed contains a type of fatty acid called linolenic acid; flaxseed is also a nonfish source of omega-3 fatty acids. The oil from flaxseed helps prevent heart attacks and strokes by its anticlotting and anti-inflammatory properties. In addition, flaxseed oil has an added positive effect on cholesterol, as it decreases LDL and raises HDL.

Flaxseeds contain substances called *lignans* along with other compounds. In the gut, bacteria convert these substances to estrogen-like compounds that may have anti-cancer effects.

Pour flaxseed oil over salads or take it by the spoonful. There are also various ways to use flaxseed oil in muffins and breads. The oil, however, should *not* be heated or cooked. Flaxseeds can be eaten whole, but they contain a shell that prevents the oil and other substances from leaving the seed and entering the gut. The seeds should, therefore, be ground.

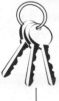

Here's to Your Heart

You can find flaxseed oil in the refrigerated section of natural-food stores. Flaxseed oil must be kept refrigerated, as it is a highly unsaturated fat and can become hydrogenated easily when exposed to heat or light! It should be kept in a dark bottle and tightly sealed. It may be stored in the freezer for up to one year, but in the refrigerator it should be used quickly.

Fish

Fish is a hot topic in the medical and nutrition communities. Many studies have demonstrated the powerful health effects of eating fish, especially in the prevention of heart disease. We know, for example, that populations with high fish consumption have a low incidence of heart attack. In addition, it's been shown that eating fish reduces the incidence of sudden death. This suggests that fish might contain a substance that lessens the effects of heart attack and stroke.

Much of the benefit of fish consumption has been through fish oil, which is an omega-3 polyunsaturated fatty acid. We discussed these fatty acids in Chapter 7, but let's briefly recap that discussion here: omega-3 fatty acids are anti-inflammatory and prevent clots. Fish oil works by substituting itself for other fatty acids in the cell membranes (and specifically in clotting cells called platelets).

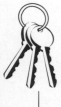

Here's to Your Heart

The best fish to eat are not lean, surprisingly. Fatty fish, such as salmon and tuna, are better for your heart, as they contain the most fish oil.

The omega fatty acids that are found in fish oils (and flaxseed oils) are good for your heart. They lower cholesterol, have a powerful antioxidant effect, and reduce the clotting ability of platelets. They also improve the health of the inner lining of the blood vessels called the endothelium. Fish oils are likely healthier than flaxseed oil; however, flaxseed oil still has anticlotting and antiatherosclerotic effects.

Fish Pills(?)

Fish oils are now available in capsular form. People who take fish oil in capsules have been shown to derive health benefits such as cholesterol reduction and especially triglyceride reduction.

However, the benefits of *eating* fish are probably greater than taking fish-oil pills. Compared with consuming fresh fish, it's been more difficult to prove that fish-oil capsules provide protection against heart disease, and not all the studies surrounding fish oils in capsule form have demonstrated healthy benefits. So here we are, back to talking about eating foods in their natural forms: it's likely better to consume fresh fish than to rely on the fish-oil capsule for health benefits. When you have a choice, then, choose fresh fish over encapsulated nutrients.

Here's to Your Heart

Dietary supplements often pale in comparison to the benefits of eating a well-balanced, nutritious diet. Many studies have shown neutral or harmful effects of various vitamins (vitamins B and E, for example) when they're used specifically as substitutes for consuming nutrients from food. Some vitamins, such as vitamin A, are highly toxic when consumed in excess (something that's nearly impossible to do when you're getting the vitamin from a food source). In addition, studies have shown that nutrients consumed from foods are more likely than supplements to reduce the incidence of certain diseases.

Olive and Canola Oils

The key to lowering cholesterol and preventing heart disease is to minimize fat consumption, especially total fat. All oils will raise cholesterol to some degree, so when you're making choices concerning what to eat, it's important to try to substitute oils with saturated fats with oils containing polyunsaturated or monounsaturated fats.

One More Time!

We talked about fat and its effect on health in Chapter 4. If you recall that discussion, we said that saturated fat is especially harmful to the blood vessels. Saturated fat is created by a process called hydrogenation, which adds hydrogen atoms to the carbon atoms of fatty acids. The hydrogenation process is detrimental for the body—it injures blood vessels! An exceptionally dangerous type of saturated fatty acid is called transfatty acids. These fatty acids are now being listed on food labels and have been linked with blood vessel damage.

Hydrogenated oils tend to remain solid at a higher temperature. For example, butter, margarine, and lard are solid at room temperature because of the hydrogenation process. Hydrogenation is highly beneficial for the food industry because it increases the shelf life of various products. Unfortunately, while food shelf life may be prolonged by adding hydrogenated fats, human life can be *reduced* by consuming hydrogenated fats.

Looking for the Best Fats

Olive oil is a polyunsaturated fat, and therefore, one of the healthier fats. (You'll remember we talked about fats are their effect on heart health in Chapter 4.) Although olive oil is low in saturated fat, the oil with the lowest saturated fat content of all the plant oils is canola oil. This should be the first oil of choice when cooking or when adding to food. In general, though, you should avoid adding oil to food whenever possible.

You can identify a food as being cholesterol-lowering by reading its nutrition label (that label located on each and every item in the grocery store). It's important to note the total number of fat grams per feed serving, the number or percentage of unsaturated fat grams, and the total number or percentage of saturated fat grams. Saturated fat is the part of the label that you should most concern yourself with when you're trying to adopt a heart-healthy diet. The lower that number is, the better!

Start looking at that saturated fat reading as a reflection of how a particular food is going to affect your LDL level. Eating foods high in saturated fat will likely raise your LDL. It's as simple as that. And even though the Paleolithic diet is ideal for the human body, your goal isn't to copy it exactly; in fact, it may be impossible to adhere to a 100 percent Paleolithic diet in this day and age. It's likely, in other words, that there will be some saturated fat creeping into your diet at some point, no matter how good you are about making healthy choices. The key, then, is to *minimize* saturated fat. One or two grams per serving are acceptable.

> **Healthy Heart Facts**
>
> The key to a heart-healthy diet is to minimize the consumption of saturated fats! Replacing vegetable oil with olive or canola oil is a step in the right direction.

The Least You Need to Know

- ◆ Soy is loaded with isoflavones and other phytoestrogens.

- ◆ Nuts contain essential fatty acids, which are good for your health!

- ◆ Flaxseed can be consumed in many different ways and is a good source of linolenic acid.

- ◆ The best fish for cardiovascular health are fatty fish because they contain the most fish oil.

- ◆ Olive and canola oils contain monounsaturated fats and are a better choice than vegetable oil or butter when cooking.

Lowering Cholesterol with Functional Foods

In This Chapter

◆ Understand how some foods provide multiple health benefits

◆ Read about foods with anticancer effects

◆ Learn about cholesterol-lowering diets

◆ Improve your health with certain beverages

◆ Know why supplements aren't usually all they're cracked up to be

With all the talk about health during the past couple of decades, people have become interested in purchasing foods that have specific health benefits. For example, it's no longer enough for many people to simply sit down and eat a well-balanced meal. They want to know what each food on the plate is going to do for them. Will this vegetable lower their blood pressure? Will this meat make them stronger? Will this whole grain improve their heart function? If one food isn't going to serve a particular function, these folks want to find another one that will.

This is quite an interesting topic, in fact, because many foods are functional foods. So if you've been eating a healthy diet, you've probably been doing your body a lot of good without even knowing it over the years!

What Are Functional Foods?

Foods that are consumed for reasons beyond their basic role as tools for survival are called *functional foods*. For the purpose of this discussion, and because it's what I recommend to my own patients, we concentrate on functional foods that are also components of the Paleolithic diet. These dietary components, as you'll recall from Chapter 7, are cholesterol-reducing and typically derived from plants.

def•i•ni•tion

Functional foods are those foods that help to improve health. These foods may lower cholesterol, reduce the incidence of cancer, prevent heart attack, or help to fight blood clots. Some functional foods, like those containing phytochemicals, are believed to have anticarcinogenic, or cancer-fighting, effects.

Phytochemicals: Fighting for Your Health

Now, what's so great about eating foods that are found in nature? Well, there are plenty of reasons. A plant-based diet reduces the incidence of heart disease and cancer. It's believed that certain substances found in plants called phytochemicals may reduce cholesterol and may also be anticarcinogenic, or cancer-fighting. Among the many types of phytochemicals are the following:

- Protease inhibitors
- Phytosterols
- Saponins
- Phenolic acids
- Phytic acid
- Isoflavones

Beta-sitosterol is a particular type of phytosterol that prevents the absorption of cholesterol from the intestine. Isoflavones, meanwhile, are similar to estrogenic steroids. As weak estrogens, they may block estrogen receptors and have antitumor activity.

Oil Try It!

Flaxseed's health benefits come from its oil, which contains alpha-linolenic acid, an omega-3 fatty acid. Flaxseed also contains lignans, which are fibrous compounds that may prevent tumor formation. Flaxseed reduces total cholesterol and LDL. Flaxseed may also provide an antiplatelet (and anticlotting) effect. Remember, clotting is one of the main mechanisms of heart attacks and strokes, so the more ways find to minimize the chances of blood clots, the better!

Carotenoids

Tomatoes contain lycopene, which is a *carotenoid*. Carotenoids are plant pigments found in various foods. Carotenoids are found in animals as well, but animals actually derive them from plants they eat.

Scientists have hypothesized that carotenoids may prevent cancer and other degenerative conditions. There is some data that a particular type of carotenoid called lutein may prevent macular degeneration, which is an age-related

def•i•ni•tion

Carotenoids may help prevent cancer and other conditions related to aging. There are three main types of carotenoids: lycopene, luteins, and beta-carotene. Common sources of carotenoids are tomatoes, broccoli, parsley, and dark leafy vegetables.

degenerative condition involving the eyes and a common age-related cause for vision loss. Interestingly, several studies have suggested that statins may also prevent macular degeneration.

Because there is no firm scientific data as to whether supplements containing carotenoids such as lutein are useful, it's recommended that you obtain carotenoids by eating foods rich in these and other substances. In other words, don't sit around just eating tomatoes; eat a well-balanced diet similar to the Paleolithic and DASH diets, both of which recommend lots of fruits and vegetables.

Healthy Heart, Unhealthy Breath

Garlic has been consumed for years for its potential cholesterol-reducing properties. In addition, garlic has been touted as having antitumor and antihypertensive (that is, blood pressure–lowering) properties. These claims have not been substantiated. However, there's also no harm in eating garlic (other than possibly offending someone with your garlicky breath), so if you just love the taste of a crushed clove or two, you might (*might*) also be doing your heart and body some good.

Healthy Foods, Healthy Benefits

Have you always turned your nose up at broccoli? Well, it's time to stop. Broccoli contains a group of compounds called glucosinolates. Indole-3-carbinol is derived from these substances and has been touted to have anti-cancer effects. At this time, there is no scientific evidence that indole-3-carbinol reduces cancer risk, but again, there's certainly no harm in testing the theory.

Although citrus fruits, such as oranges, lemons, limes, and grapefruits are good sources of vitamin C, folate, and fiber, they are also a good source of a group of compounds called limonoids, which, along with their derivatives, are being investigated for possible anti-cancer activity.

Drink Up!

Thirsty? Good. You can find healthy compounds in beverages, too. Cranberry juice, for example, is used to treat urinary tract infections in women. *E. coli* is the type of bacteria that is responsible for causing many urinary tract infections in women. *E. coli* contain structures called pili that allow for easier binding to the urinary tract. Cranberry juice may prevent certain molecules on the surface of the pili from adhering to the urinary tract and causing the subsequent urinary tract infection.

The Doctor Says

Although there are some studies linking flavonoids and polyphenols with reduced incidence of heart disease and cancer, there is no definitive data that tea—even green tea—reduces the incidence of these conditions.

Tea, meanwhile, contains substances called flavonoids and polyphenols, which have been purported to have anticancer effects. Green tea has the greatest amount of these substances.

You Get the Idea!

As I said at the beginning of this chapter, there are many, many foods that fall into the functional-food category. Vitamin D fortified milk may provides vitamin D as well as calcium. Various foods are consumed as sources of high-quality protein, such as eggs, or as a source of folic acid.

At this time, the market for functional foods is growing. People are looking for their foods to provide big health advantages, such as …

♦ Lowering cholesterol.

♦ Preventing heart disease.

♦ Preventing cancer.

One note of caution: although foods found in the produce section of the supermarket are very good for your health, the specific advertisement of functional foods for their health benefits is not regulated by any government agency in this country. Japan is the only country that has developed a specific regulatory approval process for functional foods.

> **Healthy Heart Facts**
>
> Although functional foods are not regulated in this country at this time, occasionally the government will look out for our collective health by mandating certain food requirements. The addition of folic acid to foods, for example, constitutes the fulfillment of a specific function by government agencies: to reduce to incidence of neural tube defects in infants.

How Functional Foods Work

How do functional foods help us? Generally speaking, foods that are found in nature are best for our bodies: they're low in fat, they don't contain refined sugar and carbohydrates, and they contain vitamins and minerals in their most natural forms.

As good as this sounds, there's even more that natural foods do for us: plant products contain many substances that may be protective against heart disease and cancer. However, there is no evidence that consumption of any of these compounds in isolation provides any specific benefit. You have to eat a healthy diet (instead of depending on one type of food or a supplement) to reap the benefits of healthy foods, in other words. Fish oil may be the one exception to this rule, and we'll talk about that shortly.

The most important point for you to take away from this discussion is that functional foods should be eaten for their possible protective value against various illnesses. A Paleolithic diet based upon plant products may yield cholesterol-reducing effects. Furthermore, a diet rich in plant products may protect against heart disease and also may have anticancerous effects.

I realize that the word *may* isn't definitive; however, look at the flip side of this discussion: we know for sure that consuming a diet high in fat and manmade preservatives is not good for the body. There's absolutely no harm in a diet that consists mainly of functional foods, but there is a potential for profound health benefits.

Here's to Your Heart _____

It's not possible at this time to consume individual dietary constituents, except for possibly fish oil, and expect to derive benefit from them. Functional foods work as a team, or a system, in the body. You have to eat them together to achieve the best results for your health. Studies of vitamins have also shown the importance of dietary consumption of protective compounds as part of foods (not supplements).

Working Together

There is likely a scientific explanation for why certain compounds are associated with substantial benefits when eaten in their natural forms (food, usually) over and above supplements of these same substances. Most compounds that affect human metabolism don't work in isolation. That is, you can't just eat, say, lycopene and expect to reap its health benefits. Nature doesn't work this way. Many compounds need to be taken together.

The necessity of using many compounds to prevent illness is due to the complex nature of human metabolism. In general, it's rare that an illness is caused by the absence or deficiency of a single compound. For example, vitamin-C deficiency (seen in a condition called scurvy) is rare is the United States. It's easily treated with vitamin C pills. Some diseases are caused by the absence of a single enzyme due to a genetic problem or mutation. These diseases can sometimes be treated with replacement of the one missing factor. However, most human diseases are far more complex, especially heart disease, diabetes, hypertension, abnormal cholesterol, obesity, and cancer. These illnesses are not usually due to lack of a single entity and can't be prevented or cured by supplementation of a single factor.

Healthy Heart Facts

Several years ago, the scientific community became excited when supplementation with a compound called vascular endothelial growth factor, or VEGF, showed promise in inducing the formation of new blood vessels in people with severe blockages and very sick hearts. However, the experiments did not work. It turned out that what we already knew held true here: you can't supplement with one factor and expect to grow new blood vessels.

There are so many chemical pathways and steps involved in maintaining human health that the answer to disease prevention is not likely, at least not at this time, to be found in a jar. Disease prevention is a lifelong process, ideally starting in childhood with diet and exercise. However, the good news is that it's never too late for adults—even at advanced ages—to change their lifestyles. Many scientific studies that are landmark trials in modern medicine clearly demonstrate that blood pressure reduction and cholesterol management in elderly prevents heart attacks, heart failure, and stroke, and saves lives.

Products to Look For

There are certain foods that should be absolutely be included in your diet because of the health functions they have demonstrated in major scientific studies. You'll no doubt be familiar with the main examples:

◆ Fruits

◆ Vegetables

◆ Grains

◆ Legumes

◆ Non-fat or low-fat dairy products

What do you notice about these foods? They comprise the main components of the Paleolithic diet, which reduces cholesterol, reduce blood pressure, and prevent heart disease! These foods also likely contain antioxidants and other unknown chemicals that have positive benefits on health. The best thing about the Paleolithic/functional-food diet is that it's not hard to find these foods; you need only go as far as your corner market to fill up your basket with goodness.

Keep Your Guard Up!

While you keep in mind that a balance diet is healthiest, learn to critically analyze new products that self-report their astounding health benefits. There are many supplements found in health food stores or via the Internet that are not FDA regulated! You should evaluate these types of supplements knowing that they haven't passed muster in scientific studies.

Now, this isn't sour grapes from the medical community. Indeed, just because a particular substance hasn't been proven to have health benefits up to this point doesn't preclude compounds from a plant or the synthesis of a product that may have health benefits. But one thing isn't likely to change any time soon: the natural source of a product usually yields the most health benefits.

So, for example, if you encounter a product that reports substantial health benefits, do your best to locate the source of the product. For example, if you were to encounter a plant product that has been isolated and then encapsulated, powdered, or gelatinized in the form of a pill, identify the natural source of the product—and try to go that route. It's probably better to consume the plant source of the product to reap its benefits.

Fishing for Health

Fish oils can be used to reduce high triglyceride levels. In addition, there is a growing body of scientific evidence in support of fish oils for prevention and treatment of heart disease. Of course, the best way to obtain fish oil is to eat lots of fish. Fatty fish are best, although you shouldn't take this advice to mean that you can fry up that fish and smother it with tartar sauce (both of which would add an enormous amount of saturated fat to your fish); the natural source of the fat (found in the fish oil itself) is all you need.

> **Healthy Heart Facts**
>
> Fish is best steamed or cooked in its own juices. You can also cook fish in olive oil or sunflower oil. If you're going to cook fish in oil, avoid margarine or butter and choose a mono- or unsaturated oil; also, be careful to avoid using too much oil because this can raise cholesterol.

As far as how much fish oil is good for your health … too much of anything can be harmful. If you're taking fish oil pills, you should talk to your doctor about it so that your triglyceride levels can be monitored. Remember, though, that you're far more likely to derive health benefits from the actual source of these oils—fish. When worked into a healthy Paleolithic diet, naturally derived fish oils work with other foods to improve your health.

When looking for fish-pill supplements, which actually have been shown to have some health benefits, the major products to look for will be those that contain fish oils, EPA, and DHA.

Functional Fruits

The time and money that you might spend on for which there is no sound scientific data proving a benefit in the reduction of cholesterol and heart disease would be far better spent on fruits and vegetables, which we know for a fact are beneficial to your health. Many supermarkets carry exotic fruits and vegetables; give them a try and shake things up in your diet! This is part of sticking with the Paleolithic or DASH diet, either of which helps to lower the risk for heart disease and lower cholesterol.

It's important to keep in mind that many supplements and products have been linked, one way or another (accurately or not), with health benefits and can easily be found in books, magazines, or on the Internet. Some of these products might actually be proven at some point to have some health benefits. Read the studies and keep yourself informed! If something sounds too good to be true, remember—it usually is.

In any event, it's most important to understand that many supplemental products have been linked with improved markers of disease and not actual disease prevention or reduction. Some claims may seem quite convincing, even when you do a little investigating. However, you need to search for products that demonstrate a reduction in what medical doctors call "hard endpoints," events such as heart attacks, stroke, and death. (Medical doctors know, for example, that the DASH diet plus medications reduces hard endpoints.) So focus on what's known to work for improving heart health instead of taking your chances with questionable supplements: look to maximize your potential health benefits by fruits, vegetables, whole grains, and fish.

The Least You Need to Know

♦ Functional foods may provide the body with multiple nutrients and benefits, such as lowering cholesterol.

♦ The Paleolithic diet is composed mainly of functional foods.

♦ Illness is rarely caused by one missing nutrient.

♦ There is little scientific data supporting the use of dietary supplements; a balanced, healthy diet is best for the body.

♦ Fish oils seem to be the one exception to the supplement rule, as they have shown some benefits in people who take them.

All About Omega Oils

In This Chapter

- ◆ Know how cell membranes are formed
- ◆ Understand how omega oils can help to minimize clotting and inflammation
- ◆ Learn how omega oils protect cells from oxidant damage
- ◆ Find the best sources for omega oils

Omega-3 fatty acids are powerful protective substances. They maximize the function of the membranes of important cells, such as platelets and endothelial cells (those that line the blood vessels), so that an ideal anti-inflammatory environment is created. Omega-3 polyunsaturated fatty acids modify the cell membranes of inflammatory and clotting cells, reducing atherosclerosis and the likelihood of plaque rupture. In addition, studies have shown that these fatty acids also reduce the incidence of arrhythmias (irregular heartbeats) and sudden death.

In this chapter, we get into the details of omega-3 and omega-6 fatty acids: what they do inside the body, why the work to reduce illness, and where to find them for yourself!

How to Choose Them

When we refer to omega-6 and omega-3 acids as being essential, that means they're used in the body; however, the body cannot produce these acids, so we have to ingest them from food sources.

Cell membranes are necessary for the transmission of signals from one cell to another, for integrated function of tissues and organs, and for various other functions. All cell membranes are made up of lipids, or fats. These essential fatty acids are required for the construction of lipid components of cells. As a result, lipids are required—or essential—for life, because cells can't exist or function without their membranes.

Healthy Heart Facts

Cell membranes are composed of a double layer of lipid molecules. One end of the lipid molecule attracts water; the other side repels water. This is why oil and water do not mix. Oil is insoluble in water. Triglycerides, oils, and fats are lipid compounds that do not mix with water. As a result, lipid molecules make ideal cell membranes. They keep the cell contents inside and the exterior stuff outside.

For other molecules to cross the lipid membrane, they must pass through pores that are lined with charged proteins that will allow some compounds in and keep others out. Frequently, these proteins have sugar molecules attached that help the proteins on the cell membrane communicate with neighboring cells. This is how cells interact with each other.

Essential for Interaction

All cells interact. Nerves cells must interact to conduct nerve impulses. Heart cells must interact to conduct the electricity of the heart and for the heart to beat as a unit. Inflammatory cells must interact to draw more inflammatory cells to an area where germs are located or where cholesterol is being deposited or where cholesterol plaques are rupturing. The health of the blood clotting elements (such as platelets) is partly dependent on the health of the platelet membrane, and the health of the platelet membrane is partly dependent upon the lipids that make up the membrane.

When the lipids of the cell membrane contain omega-3 and omega-6 fatty acids, platelets are healthier and are less likely to clot. When the platelet membranes contain more omega-3 and omega-6 fatty acids, the blood vessels are more likely to dilate. This is because the platelet membranes construct substances called *prostaglandins* that can either dilate or constrict blood vessels. When there are more omega-3 fatty acids in the membranes than other fatty acids, there are more prostaglandins that open up the blood vessels, which prevent blood clotting, are anti-inflammatory, and prevent plaque rupture and heart attacks.

def•i•ni•tion

Prostaglandins are substances that either dilate (open) or constrict blood vessels. Omega-3 fatty acids in the membranes of platelets create a situation in which there are more dilatory prostaglandins present. This reduces the risk of blood clots and prevents plaque rupture and heart attacks.

Oxidants are normal products of human metabolism. Because they contain charged compounds, they are unstable and capable of doing harm to cell membranes. **Antioxidants,** such as omega-3 fatty acids, work to stop oxidant damage. **Free radicals** are one type of oxidant.

Essential for Antioxidation

Antioxidants prevent damage to the cell membranes. *Oxidants* are intermediates in metabolism that have the ability to damage the cell membranes. Oxidants are charged elements with extra electrons; they are therefore unstable and capable of doing harm inside the body by chemically damaging the integrity of the cell membranes. Omega-3 fatty acids help prevent oxidation induced damage to cell membranes.

Omega-3 oils have protective effects against cancer and heart disease. The lipid that makes up the membranes of cells can be easily damaged. Various oxidative substances called *free radicals* can destroy lipids and render them dangerous to the body. Free radicals are charged compounds that act like bleach. These charged compounds can cause the lipids to become charged as well.

The Doctor Says

The process wherein molecules become oxidized renders them more likely to be able to cause adverse effects within cells. For instance, oxidation of lipids increases the chance for formation of atherosclerotic plaques and increases risk for heart attack.

Fishy Sources of Omega-3

Interestingly, a good source of omega-3 fatty acids is whale blubber, a staple of the Eskimos' diet. The incidence of heart disease is very low among Eskimos despite their high-fat diet because their diet contains high concentrations of omega-3 fatty acids. Their platelets and endothelial cells (the cells that line the inside of blood vessels) have omega-3 fatty acids substituted for other fatty acids. This produces a protective antiatherosclerotic effect and an anticlotting effect.

There are principally two omega-3 fatty acids that are derived from fish oil and that can be either consumed directly from fish or via fish oil supplements. The two fatty acids are called EPA (eicosapentaenoic acid) and DHA (docosatetraenoic acid). They can be combined in pill form twice a day. The total daily dose is 3 grams.

Aside from whale blubber and supplements, excellent sources of omega-3 fatty acids include flaxseed oil and certain types of fish, including the following:

Healthy Heart Facts
The only real side effect of fish-oil supplements is a fishy taste or scent. Often, people complain of "fishy burps" when using these substances. Some of the names for these pills are Promega, Cardio-Mega 3, Marine Lipid Concentrate, MaxEPA, and SuperEPA 1200.

- Mackerel
- Salmon
- Halibut
- Trout
- Herring

Spiny dogfish, sardines, pilchards, tuna, sturgeon, anchovies, sprats, bluefish, and mullet are also good sources of omega-3.

Omega-3 as an Anti-Inflammatory

Fish oil also works to lessen the effects of pro-clotting compounds in the blood. This process is a bit complex, so I've broken it down, point by point:

- Inflammatory and anti-inflammatory compounds are made from components called arachidonic acid, which are found in the membranes of platelets (clotting cells).
- Arachidonic acid undergoes a complex process where various enzymes convert into inflammatory and anti-inflammatory lipids. One of these lipids is called thromboxane.

   ◆ One particular type of thromboxane formed is called thromboxane A_2; this compound activates platelets and causes them to stick to each other and form blood clots. It also constricts blood vessels. Thromboxane A_2 is inflammatory.

   ◆ Fish oil, meanwhile, can integrate itself into lipids in the membranes of the platelets. (Remember, all cell membranes are made up of lipids.) When thromboxane is formed from lipids that contain omega-3 fatty acids, the thromboxane formed is thromboxane A_3, which is less pro-clotting and less inflammatory than thromboxane A_2.

As a result of the omega-3 fatty acids in the platelet membranes, any reaction is less inflammatory. And as you already know, inflammation plays a key role in plaque rupture.

Omega-6

Although we need both omega-6 and omega-3 fatty acids in our diet, people consume an excess of omega-6 fatty acids. Neither type of fatty acid increases LDL and total cholesterol, but they each have different affects on cell membrane integrity and function. As a result of their diverse functions inside the body, omega-6 and omega-3 fatty acids have different effects on the incidences of heart attacks, strokes, cancers and other illnesses.

The difference between omega-3 and omega-6 fatty acids lies where the double bond is located in the fat molecule. If you remember our discussion of the formation of fats from Chapter 2, you'll recall that fatty acids are long chains of carbon atoms with hydrogen attached. Omega-3 fatty acids have a double bond at the third carbon atom in the chain. Omega-6 fatty acids have a double bond at the sixth position. I don't expect you to re-create this in your home laboratory; the important thing for you to know is that the location of the double bond is important to the makeup and function of the cell membranes. Where that double-bond occurs affects the function of the fatty acid.

Healthy Ratios

Omega-6 fatty acids are found the following oils, among others:

   ◆ Safflower   ◆ Sesame

   ◆ Sunflower   ◆ Hemp

   ◆ Corn   ◆ Pumpkin

◆ Soybean

◆ Walnut

◆ Wheat germ

◆ Evening primrose

Here's to Your Heart

When using flaxseed oil or fish oil, be careful not to expose these oils to heat. Heating oil adds hydrogen atoms to it. This process destroys omega-3 oils and renders them less effective as antioxidants.

Omega-6 fatty acids are also found in baked goods, cereals, eggs, animal meats, poultry, margarine, and vegetable oils, which explains why their levels have risen dramatically in the past 100 years or so. Although the omega-6 fatty acids are essential, the ratio of omega-6 to omega-3 is important to obtain the proper ratio within the cell membranes to achieve ideal cell membrane integrity and function. The ideal ratio of omega-6 to omega-3 is likely to be 3 or 4 to 1, not 10 or 20 to 1 as it is in Western diets.

How to Use Them

The omega-3 fatty acids (fish oil), can be derived from dietary sources or from supplements. There is some controversy within the medical literature as to the benefit of tablets for prevention of heart disease. In general, the data appears favorable as far as fish-pill supplements are concerned.

The data, however, is not nearly as powerful for fish oil as it is for aspirin as an anti-clotting drug or as a protective agent against heart attack. In addition, the data for the beneficial effects are not nearly as powerful for fish as for the cholesterol-lowering drugs called statins. Fish oil can be used as an ancillary drug, used in conjunction with other medications, especially for elevated triglycerides.

The Least You Need to Know

◆ Cell membranes are composed of lipids.

◆ Platelets are responsible for inflammation and clotting in the body, including inside the blood vessels.

◆ Omega-3 and omega-6 can substitute themselves in platelet cell membranes, reducing inflammatory reactions and clotting.

◆ Fish is an excellent source of omega oils.

◆ Fish-oil supplements also provide health benefits.

Chapter 11

Drinking to Your Health

In This Chapter

- ◆ Learn about alcohol usage and heart health
- ◆ Read about the studies that led to the idea that alcohol might improve health
- ◆ Understand the difference between scientific and observational studies
- ◆ Educate yourself on what moderate really means
- ◆ Learn about safer alternatives improving your cardiovascular health

Alcohol consumption has a narrow spectrum and limited role in our health. Moderate alcohol consumption has been associated with a reduction in heart disease in observational studies. However, despite these findings the publicity they've generated, there are much better and safer ways to improve your heart's health.

This chapter discusses the flaws that surround observational studies. Just realize for now that while the effects of drinking on the heart may be beneficial, we simply don't know beyond the shadow of a doubt that this is true. This chapter also takes you through the ins and outs of the theoretical benefits of moderate alcohol consumption and also points out some of the possible hazards of crossing the line between moderate and excessive drinking.

The French Paradox

The French are one group of people who have experienced a reduction in the incidence of heart disease with light to moderate alcohol intake. The *French paradox* refers to this relatively low incidence of heart disease in a population that also consumes a diet rather high in fat and calories. (It's so hard not to hate them, *oui*?)

No one is truly certain why some populations have less heart disease than others. However, there appears to be a north-south gradient of heart disease risk in Europe. That is, the northern countries (such as Finland) have a higher risk for heart disease than do the southern countries, such as Spain and France. This north-south division has been seen with other diseases, also, such as multiple sclerosis, lupus, and various diseases that are thought to be due to infections.

Now, this infection connection is interesting because there is a theory that holds that certain infectious diseases may be triggers for heart attacks: there are increased incidences of heart attacks during the flu season and during the cold months. Also, various bacteria have been found within cholesterol plaques inside of heart arteries. There are no clear explanations for any of these observations at this time.

The Top-Secret French Fat-and-Alcohol Diet

The French always seem to be coming up with some hot new diet that eludes the rest of the world. Why is it that French women don't get fat? How is it that these people drink wine and eat croissants and stay rather healthy? What are they doing that we aren't?

The reduced incidence of heart disease in the French has been attributed—at least in part—to their higher alcohol consumption. Observational studies have noted a decrease in the incidence and mortality of heart disease in French populations who consume alcohol in moderation. However, this is not a diet that we should try to copy, tempting as it may seem. One reason why observational studies are flawed and give us flawed results is that the populations at the outset of the studies differ in ways that are unknown.

To put this simply: it is not advisable to increase your caloric consumption and dietary fat intake simply because you consume alcohol in light to moderate quantities. More importantly, you cannot use light-to-moderate alcohol consumption to medicate a diet high in calories or fats simply because of what the French paradox seems to be telling us—because for *most* people, a diet high in fat and calories will result in cardiovascular disease.

Healthy Heart Facts

Observational studies, such as the French paradox, are often flawed. Another famously flawed study called the Nurses Health Study revealed that women who took estrogen-replacement therapy had a lower incidence of heart disease, but we know now that this just isn't so. It's believed that the erroneous result from the Nurses Health Study was due to a difference in the women who took estrogen-replacement therapy versus those who did not. In other words, women who took estrogen-replacement therapy were likely more health conscious than women in the general population. Because these women were, in general, more health oriented, they took better care of themselves in terms of other risk factors, such as diet and exercise as well as taking other medications, which may explain their heart healthiness.

Defining Moderate Intake

There's more to defining moderate than simply spelling out the meaning of the word (however, we do that in this section, anyway). To understand where the idea that moderate alcohol intake leads to a healthier heart, we need to first take a deeper look at the kind of studies that gave us this information in the first place.

We already mentioned that there's a serious problem with relying on data from observational studies. In this section, we explain why in a more complete manner. It's important for you to understand that there isn't any hard scientific evidence that links alcohol usage and heart health, and it's actually not even possible to gather that kind of information. (You're dying to know why, right? Read on...)

A Word on Observational Studies

Observational studies are *not* strictly scientific studies. These studies follow a group of individuals over time and compare that group with a similar group that differs with respect to the variable that is being studied. So in the case of observational studies that suggest that alcohol may reduce heart-disease risk, populations of drinkers were compared with populations of nondrinkers over time. It was noted that the drinkers had a lower incidence of heart disease than the nondrinkers. Only the drinkers who drank lightly to moderately had benefits.

These studies had many problems. First, because observational studies are not truly scientific, they often lead to erroneous information. To conduct a scientific study, you have to take two identical groups of people who differ in only one respect—the variable (or study item being looked at in the study). The groups should then be followed over time to see what happens to them with respect to some predetermined outcome.

For example, a scientific study would look at 1,000 heart-attack survivors with LDL cholesterol levels greater than 160 mg/dl and give half of them a cholesterol-lowering drug and the other half a drug that *looks* like a cholesterol-lowering drug (called a placebo) and then observe them for at least six months to determine what percentage experience a decrease in LDL and what percentage experience a decrease in second heart attacks. Neither the subject nor the doctors giving the drug know whether the pills are the actual drug or the placebo. This is a scientific experiment. These types of studies were actually conducted to determine whether cholesterol-reducing medications called statins actually reduce cholesterol and heart attacks. These studies showed that statins reduce cholesterol and heart attacks and form the basis for modern therapy to reduce cholesterol and heart attacks in people with elevated or even normal cholesterol levels.

Sounds complicated, right? Well, conducting a scientific experiment *is* complicated, but that's why the results we get from them are usually so accurate. These types of rigorous studies were *not* done with alcohol. However, there does seem to be some evidence—as we see with the French paradox—that alcohol in moderate amounts may benefit the heart. We talk more about drinking in moderation later in this chapter.

A Placebo Beer, Please

One reason why rigorous *scientific* studies were not conducted on the effects of alcohol consumption on the heart is that these types of studies cannot be done. You just can't take two groups of people and give half of them alcohol and the other half a drink that resembles alcohol, for several reasons:

◆ First, those subjects not receiving alcohol will know that they have received a placebo. Likewise, the group that has received the alcohol will know they have received the alcohol.

◆ Second, it's likely to be difficult to control the amount of alcohol consumed by each subject.

◆ Third, and most important, it's unethical to administer alcohol to test subjects.

The best scientific experiments on this subject can merely observe populations of people who consume alcohol versus those who do not. The problem with these observational studies, of course, is that these studies have revealed the wrong answer many times. So we have no real way of knowing whether alcohol has a positive effect on heart health, or whether other factors come into play and make it appear as though alcohol is beneficial to the cardiovascular system. Either way, light-to-moderate alcohol consumption doesn't seem to be harmful (as long as you don't have any health problems that dictate your abstaining from alcohol).

In Theory...

In contrast to the lack of rigorous scientific information on the role of alcohol in heart disease prevention, there are *theoretical* benefits that come from light-to-moderate alcohol consumption:

◆ First, the populations of individuals who consume alcohol lightly to moderately have a reduced incidence of heart disease.

◆ Secondly (and again, theoretically), alcohol increases HDL. In reality, however, this may not be a beneficial effect because there are safer ways to increase HDL. One example of a safer way to increase HDL is exercise. Another way to increase HDL is medication, such as with a fibric acid or a statin.

◆ Another theoretical beneficial effect of alcohol is that it reduces the ability of platelets (the clotting cells in the blood) to form a blood clot. A decreased likelihood of platelet clotting is likely to lead to a reduced incidence of heart attacks and strokes.

These effects sound pretty good, but they're tempered by the fact that at this point, the benefits of alcohol have not been proven.

The Meaning of Moderate

The current recommendation from scientists is that it's permissible to consume alcohol in light to moderate amounts. *Moderate alcohol consumption* is defined as one to two drinks per day for a male and one drink per day for a female.

def•i•ni•tion

Moderate alcohol consumption refers to the consumption of one to two drinks per day for a man and one drink per day for a woman. A drink is defined as a 12-ounce beer, 6 ounces of wine, or 1¼ to 1½ ounces of liquor. Approximately seven drinks per week are considered moderate.

If you don't drink now, *don't start* in an effort to improve your heart's health. No one should *begin* to consume alcohol to achieve any health benefits. Although alcohol may increase HDL levels, it isn't recommended for health benefits or for preventing or treating cardiovascular disease! What this moderate intake really means is that if someone is *already* consuming alcohol in light to moderate amounts, it does not have to be discontinued unless there are other adverse health conditions that make *not* drinking advisable.

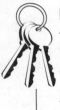

Here's to Your Heart

There has been much controversy and discussion over the purported benefits of alcohol consumption relative to its source over the years. If there are benefits to alcohol consumption, there is no scientific evidence that there is any benefit regarding the source of the alcohol. In other words, it doesn't matter whether you drink red wine, white wine, beer, or hard alcohol as long as you stay within the moderate limits.

Alcohol Is No Substitute for a Healthy Lifestyle

There are multiple proven (and safe) alternatives to alcohol consumption for people who are interested in cholesterol reduction but who are not necessarily interested in a glass of chardonnay or a bottle of beer. You already know what they are: increasing exercise activity, improving your diet, and taking cholesterol-reducing medication, such as fibric acid and statins.

Word of Warning

Alcohol consumed in amounts exceeding what we'd call moderate actually increases the risk for heart disease. In fact, alcohol is a powerful poison to heart and skeletal muscle. Various experiments have shown that alcohol causes a weakening of heart muscle in a dose-response relationship. In other words, the more alcohol someone consumes, the greater the weakening and toxicity of the heart muscle.

Alcohol is one of the most common causes of a dilated cardiomyopathy, which is the type of heart-muscle weakness (and heart failure) a person develops from causes other than blockages in the heart blood vessels and high blood pressure.

More Not-So-Glowing Reviews for Alcohol

Although alcohol has been associated with a reduced incidence for heart disease, because of the way the studies have been conducted, the data is confusing. Even the advice your doctor gives you is likely to be less-than-precise: we tell people that less than one drink per day is not likely to help their hearts and more than two per day is detrimental. Because alcohol is habit forming and dangerous in other respects, it is *not* a good idea to advise people to drink. Binge drinking increases risk.

Below are more warnings that you might hear in your doctor's office concerning alcohol and your health:

- We usually advise patients to stop drinking if their triglycerides are elevated. Alcohol definitely raises triglycerides.

- Alcohol is a frequent cause of high blood pressure. Elevated blood pressure and high cholesterol are powerful synergistic risk factors that increase risk for heart attack together, so we advise patients whose blood pressure is even a few millimeters elevated to abstain or cut back.

- Alcohol is believed to elevate HDL. However, there are various subfractions of HDL. Alcohol might not elevate the beneficial subfractions and might elevate the unbeneficial subfractions instead.

Alcohol is also a leading cause for heart muscle arrhythmias, or irregular heartbeats. There is a common arrhythmia associated with alcohol consumption called *atrial fibrillation*. This arrhythmia is frequently seen in emergency rooms around the holiday season (when nondrinkers are more likely to be consuming alcohol), hence its nickname, Holiday Heart Syndrome. Excess alcohol consumption can trigger this irregular heartbeat that increases one's risk for stroke dramatically.

Atrial fibrillation is a leading cause for stroke. Furthermore, high blood pressure is also a leading cause for stroke. High blood pressure, as said earlier, is often caused by alcohol. So excess drinking can cause multiple adverse conditions, and increases your risk for stroke significantly.

The Doctor Says

Alcohol is really a toxin. It's broken down by the liver into various compounds that are toxic to the liver as well as other organs. Alcohol is a toxin for both heart muscle and skeletal muscle and causes thousands of cases of cardiomyopathy, or heart failure.

Because alcohol is toxic to many organs, it's a powerful *carcinogen*. Alcohol, in fact, is one leading cause of preventable cancer in the United States. It's especially carcinogenic when combined with other cancer-causing substances, such as cigarettes. In addition, when alcohol and tobacco smoking are combined, a person's cardiovascular risk shoots up, as tobacco smoking is a powerful risk factor for heart disease and alcohol elevates blood pressure.

def•i•ni•tion

A **carcinogen** is a substance that can cause cancer. Alcohol and cigarettes are known carcinogens, and as unhealthy as they are individually, when used together, their carcinogenic effects are synergistic. That is, they work together to increase your risk of developing cancer!

To sum up: while alcohol in moderation may do your heart some good, drinking to excess certainly won't do anything but harm to your heart and the rest of your body. So use your good sense and your best judgment and keep your alcohol usage to a minimum.

The Least You Need to Know

◆ There is limited data that links alcohol and heart disease prevention.

◆ Alcohol increases triglyceride levels in the bloodstream.

◆ Alcohol should not be used to compensate for a high-calorie and high-fat diet.

◆ Exercise, diet, and medications are still more effective ways to lower cholesterol.

Chapter 12

Caffeine and Your Heart

In This Chapter

- ◆ Why coffee is no longer withheld from heart attack patients
- ◆ Learn about the side effects of caffeine
- ◆ Read about the antioxidant effects of tea
- ◆ Get a handle on irregular heartbeats that may be caused by caffeine

Coffees and teas have been around for thousands of years and are some of the most commonly consumed beverages worldwide. You may consider yourself something of a coffee connoisseur, craving that first drop of caffeine before you've even opened your eyes in the morning. But if you're a person who's been diagnosed with heart disease, is it safe to sip that cup of Joe? Haven't you heard somewhere that coffee is bad for the heart?

Well, you did hear that news correctly: years ago, coffee was on a list of restricted substances for heart patients. However, in the last two decades, there has been a loosening in the restrictions regarding caffeinated beverages for people with heart trouble. In this chapter, we'll discuss the possible health benefits and potential drawbacks of consuming caffeine.

Caffeine Fix!

Coffees and teas contain many chemical compounds, many of which, believe it or not, are unknown to us. What we do know is that one of the primary reasons people drink coffee and tea is for the effects of the caffeine component. Caffeine, as you probably know, is a mild stimulant.

For the most part, caffeine is harmless—at least in the quantities that are present in a cup of coffee or tea. However, if you have a heart condition or are concerned about your cardiovascular health, consult your physician about your caffeine intake before consuming or continuing your regular consumption of coffee or tea.

> **Healthy Heart Facts**
>
> Coffee and tea are under the scientific microscope regarding their possible health benefits. Both beverages contain bioactive components which are being studied to determine their effects on cholesterol, the heart, and cancer.

Maybe you wonder why caffeine provides a burst of energy. Specific receptors in the body, including inside the heart, respond to caffeine. To give you a clearer picture of what happens when caffeine meets these receptors, we need to take a detour through the emergency room.

The caffeine receptors inside the body also respond to medications with similar chemical structures; these medications, it will come as no surprise, produce effects similar to those of caffeine. One of these medications, called theophylline, is used to treat asthma in children and is frequently administered as an intravenous infusion for an emergency asthma attack. One of the side effects of theophylline is heart palpitations and a rapid heart rate. This medication releases a powerful substance in the body called adenosine that causes blood vessels to dilate, which in turn allows blood to flow more effectively. Sometimes pure adenosine is given intravenously for severe, in-hospital rapid heart actions.

Back to your morning coffee. Caffeine works by releasing adenosine inside the body. After a cup of coffee or tea, your blood vessels dilate and you feel your heart rate increase.

Caffeine and Cholesterol

Coffee likely does not have any significant effect on cholesterol. When people make dietary choices, they should focus their energy on avoiding foods that clearly have adverse effects on cholesterol. There is little to be gained from limiting coffee consumption or modifying it dramatically. If you require a morning cup of coffee to start the day, the quality-of-life issues associated with your little pick-me-up first thing in the morning are likely to outweigh any significant adverse effects.

There may be some people who experience particular cardiac arrhythmias or sensitivities to caffeine. Anyone who has a documented health condition for which their physician has advised them to avoid caffeine should follow the advice of their physician. In general, though, the caffeine-avoidance recommendations for cardiac patients in the past have been overrated. People with heart disease should focus their energy on taking their medications following the dietary and exercise advice of their physicians.

> **The Doctor Says**
>
> Caffeine usually isn't a contributing risk factor for cholesterol or heart disease. You're likely to experience far greater benefits by following the advice of a physician regarding diet, exercise, and various medications, including those that reduce cholesterol, than you'll experience by cutting coffee out of your diet.

The Lowdown on That Cup of Joe

So far as we know, caffeine does not have any major beneficial or detrimental effects on either the blood vessels or other organs. Typically, 15 or 20 years ago, when someone was admitted to the critical care unit with a heart attack, caffeine was generally withheld. In fact, various other things were withheld, such as early ambulation (getting up and out of bed), which today are actually advisable! Caffeine was withheld due to a belief that it was a stimulant and triggered certain potentially lethal *arrhythmias* that could lead to sudden death after a heart attack. We now know that this is not true. Caffeine use after a heart attack is no longer contraindicated.

PVCs

Having just given you the general recommendation concerning heart patients and caffeine, I'm going to narrow this down a bit. Some people are sensitive to the effects of caffeine; in these people, caffeine may trigger an *arrhythmia*. Most caffeine-induced arrhythmias are benign. Sometimes, young people may experience premature beats called *premature ventricular contractions (PVCs)* or premature atrial contractions.

> **def•i•ni•tion**
>
> An **arrhythmia** is an abnormal heartbeat. There are several different forms of arrhythmias; some are lethal, and others are relatively harmless. Caffeine-induced **arrhythmias,** such as **premature ventricular contractions (PVCs)** are generally benign.

These PVCs were quite misunderstood years ago and were believed to be a harbinger for sudden death. PVCs were thought to trigger lethal arrhythmias (such as ventricular tachycardia or ventricular fibrillation, both of which can be deadly). As a result, cardiologists used to give medications to suppress these PVCs, suspecting that the suppression of these PVCs would decrease the risk for sudden death. This was especially widely practiced in individuals who had recently experienced a heart attack. In fact, individuals admitted to the hospital with or without PVCs were routinely administered an intravenous drip of a chemical to prevent these PVCs. Basically, all cardiologists attempted to suppress PVCs. This was part of the withholding-coffee rationale.

> **Healthy Heart Facts**
>
> The PVC story serves to affirm how critically important it is to perform rigorous scientific studies before beginning a therapy. Although implementing a therapy may seem attractive on first examination, it needs to be tested scientifically. This lesson has been relearned multiple times under various scenarios.

However, in the early 1990s, a major shift in thinking occurred. Several large studies determined that the medications that doctors gave to patients with these extra beats were increasing their chances of death! The medications were decreasing the PVCs but harming patients in the interim. These studies were so powerful that the entire PVC hypothesis was disposed of.

We'll talk a little bit more about different types of arrhythmias and their relation to caffeine later in this chapter.

It's What's in the Coffee That Counts!

In general, drinking coffee isn't associated with any adverse effects. The studies on the benefits and risks of coffee do not yield any substantial effects. If you require a cup or coffee (or even a few cups of coffee) in the morning, you're unlikely to incur significant

> **The Doctor Says**
>
> Although caffeine appears to be safe for heart patients, many regular coffee drinkers find that they suffer from headaches when they skip their java in the morning. This is one minor side effect of kicking a caffeine habit; headaches can be reduced by cutting back on caffeine gradually.

adverse health effects—unless you have a documented cardiac arrhythmia or sensitivity to caffeine. As with all dietary choices, moderation is the key!

Although the effects of caffeine seem to be completely benign, you should be careful about what you're adding to your coffee. Do not add sugar. Also, ideally, you should drink your coffee black because creamers tend to be high in fat and calories. A few creamers in moderation are unlikely to be associated with any significant fat consumption. Low-calorie creamers are better than whole cream or creamers made with partially hydrogenated fats. Avoid coffees that are purchased in coffee houses and that contain whipped cream, sugar, various high-calorie syrups, and flavorings—although they're delicious, they tend to be high in calories and fat.

Green Tea

Green tea comes from plant species called *Camellia sinensis*. When comparing green tea to black tea, green tea is the healthier as it is unoxidized. Let's talk about this process for a moment.

When the body metabolizes various compounds and conducts its daily activities of producing energy from food, various intermediate products of metabolism are formed that may be toxic. These compounds are often called *free radicals*, or charged molecules. These charged compounds have extra electrons, giving them a negative charge. They are usually very reactive, chemically seeking to become uncharged. These charged compounds may cause damage to cells. For instance, they may affect the cell membrane in such a way that the membrane is damaged and cannot perform its functions of communicating with other cells.

The body has a defense system against oxidants composed of molecules called *antioxidants* that neutralize the oxidants produced in normal metabolism. As a result, the cell is protected. Antioxidants exist at the same level of cell formation that is responsible for producing the oxidants in the first place; for this reason, the oxidants are rapidly degraded before they can cause significant damage.

The Doctor Says

Oxidants can cause cell damage and also damage the DNA (genes within the nucleus of cells), causing mutations and other types of cell damage. This can lead to cancers. **Antioxidants** work to prevent this type of damage. **Free radicals** are one type of oxidant.

Green Tea and Phytochemicals

Over time, excessive oxidants can lead to the progression of atherosclerosis. Oxidants are powerful proatherosclerotic compounds. In addition to stimulating the chronic deposition of cholesterol on the inside of arteries, they participate in plaque rupture by causing inflammatory cells to infiltrate the region of the plaque. As a result, oxidants can lead to heart attacks.

Green tea has been shown to contain various plant chemicals called phytochemicals that may provide an antioxidant effect; these effects have been demonstrated in laboratory experiments. Although the consumption of these phytochemicals and other antioxidants makes intuitive sense and although the data appears promising, it's a little too early to recommend the consumption of green tea as an antioxidant.

All recommendations to consume particular dietary constituents for health benefits should be associated with scientific studies that prove benefits. Currently, the scientific data is lacking in the form rigorous scientific studies.

Both green and black teas have multiple substances that may improve cholesterol levels and improve health. Green tea is likely to be the healthier of the two. Studies have shown beneficial effects on cholesterol levels and measures of oxidation when green and black teas are consumed. However, there are no definitive studies in the literature proving a benefit in terms of improved cholesterol levels and reduction of heart disease or cancer in people who consume these beverages.

Those last two sentences may seem to contradict each other, but it's really a matter of the amount of research that's been done: the studies in the medical literature have suggested that there may be benefit to consumption of green tea. Green tea has been associated with possible beneficial effects on cholesterol and its metabolism in laboratory experiments. Some human studies are suggestive of a possible benefit. However, large, scientifically conducted studies have not been conducted. The green tea studies are hypothesis-generating but not any higher.

Black Tea

Black tea, like green tea, comes from the species *C. sinensis*. Black tea has antioxidants and compounds that are beneficial, in theory, for blood vessels and as anti-inflammatory compounds.

There are no definitive studies in the medical literature at this time substantiating a benefit for black tea in terms of reduction in cholesterol, or the incidence of heart disease or cancer. It is possible that over time, substances may be isolated from black and green teas that may have therapeutic benefit. When one considers that penicillin, which revolutionized modern medicine, was derived from a fungus, it is not inconceivable that various plants may yield powerful substances that will improve the health of humans.

How to Take It

There have been studies done to look at coffee consumption based upon the number of cups a person drinks per day. One of these studies, completed in 2005, reviewed over 100 previous coffee studies (this was a study of the studies, if you will). The final report showed no increase in risk for heart disease with coffee consumption.

Some studies have shown a decrease in the risk of type 2 diabetes in people who consume more than five cups of coffee per day, when compared to people who drink fewer than two cups per day. In addition, it is likely that filtered coffee has a better effect on LDL and other cholesterol components than boiled coffee, which may actually increase LDL. There is no consensus in the medical literature about coffee's effect on LDL.

Furthermore, no guidelines have been issued from major scientific societies, although caffeine is no longer contraindicated post heart attack.

Potential Side Effects

Coffee may produce side effects in people who have certain heart rhythm disorders that predispose them to an increased risk of arrhythmias, or irregular heartbeats. Let's discuss the heart rhythm for a moment.

The heart creates its own electricity. This electricity is used to stimulate the heart to beat or squeeze on a regular basis. Normally, the heart has a certain rhythm of beating, like a drum. It usually beats 60 to 100 times per minute, regularly, day in, day out.

The electricity that creates the heartbeat moves from the top of the heart to the bottom and percolates through the walls of the heart. If the heartbeat or rhythm changes speed to slower than 60 or faster than 100, it has an arrhythmia, or abnormal heartbeat. Sometimes, the heartbeat can be irregular or there may be a series of rapid beats. If the late beats start in the bottom of the heart, this may indicate a dangerous rhythm problem, such as ventricular tachycardia. Ventricular tachycardia can degenerate into ventricular fibrillation, which is terminal.

An early beat is called a premature beat. A premature beat can arise from the top of the heart or the bottom. Coffee may increase the frequency of these premature beats or trigger their onset. Normally, healthy hearts have a few of these early beats. Coffee can increase their frequency and make them noticeable to the individual; however, normally, the premature beats are imperceptible. (Doctors may tell their patients to avoid coffee if it's associated with frequent early beats that are perceptible.) Perceptible early beats may provoke anxiety. Sometimes, medication can be used to decrease the perceptibility of the premature beats, but often, the side effects of the medication are more troublesome than the premature beats' perceptibility. For this reason, it is often best not to treat the premature beats, especially if they are benign.

> ### Healthy Heart Facts
>
> Premature beats can be a harbinger of heart disease. Premature beats may be dangerous if the heart muscle is damaged by a previous heart attack, or is weakened, but only if there are groups of them.

Unless you have been specifically diagnosed with an irregular heartbeat like those I've described above, moderate caffeine consumption will not harm your heart.

Coffees and teas may have beneficial effects, and except for those individuals for whom caffeine is contraindicated (and this is uncommon), there are few side effects to coffee and tea consumption. You can most likely consume these beverages in moderation with the knowledge that the likelihood of major cardiovascular side effects is low.

The Least You Need to Know

- Coffee is no longer contraindicated for people who have had heart attacks.

- There are no major known side effects of caffeine.

- It's unlikely that caffeine has any substantial beneficial effects in terms of cholesterol reduction or reduction in the incidence of heart disease and cancer.

- There may be compounds that have potent actions that are yet to be isolated from these coffee and tea.

Chapter 13

Putting It All Together

In This Chapter

- ◆ Reduce cholesterol with the three-pronged approach
- ◆ Read how you can stick with a healthy diet
- ◆ Understand how other people make exercise a part of their daily routine
- ◆ Advice for sticking with a healthy diet

The key to lowering cholesterol is following a three-pronged approach for lowering LDL and raising HDL. The three components of this program are sticking to a low-fat diet, getting involved with an enjoyable form of exercise, and using medications appropriately when indicated. The combination of all three factors will lower cholesterol and reduce the incidence of heart disease.

Listen to what your doctor has to say, and then look to the tips outlined in this book to decrease your cholesterol and your risk for heart disease and other illnesses. We talk more about using medication for lowering cholesterol in Part 4 of this book; this chapter talks specifically about how to incorporate diet and activity into your daily routine.

Developing a Lifelong Eating Program

The key to a lifelong healthy eating program is the maintenance of good eating habits. After you've implemented good eating habits, the major risk is the resumption of previous poor eating habits.

Giving up your favorite high-fat foods may seem like an impossible task at this point. Most adults who eat unhealthy foods on a regular basis have developed their eating habits and preferences over a long period of time (often over an entire lifetime). If you've never eaten fish without the beer-battered, deep-fried coating, for example, you'll note that that the texture and flavor of grilled, broiled, or baked fish is quite different. Likewise with vegetables: minus the cheese sauce and butter, broccoli and cauliflower have their own unique tastes.

Enjoying healthy foods is just a matter of getting used to foods in their most natural states, something we talked about in greater detail in Chapter 7.

Here's to Your Heart

The Paleolithic diet advocates consuming foods that are found in nature—low-fat meats, vegetables, fruits, and whole grains. Starting a low-fat diet initially may lower HDL, as fat is needed to manufacture HDL. Later, the HDL may rise. It's possible that different HDL subcomponents may be affected by the implementation of a low-fat diet. In other words, the decrease in HDL experienced when a low-fat diet is started may reflect a decrease in nonprotective or less protective HDL components.

It's human nature to revert to previous, lifelong, and learned behaviors, such as eating unhealthy foods. Doctors understand that it's difficult to overhaul your lifestyle and cut back on fat. Eating a healthy diet isn't a recommendation that we give out flippantly, thinking that it should be a piece of cake (angel food if you must, as it's lowest in fat). However, sticking with a low-fat diet is necessary for heart health, which makes the struggle to stay on the straight and narrow worth it in the long run.

Willpower!

Developing and adhering to a lifelong healthy eating program requires vigilance and willpower. It may seem logical that the initial cut-down on fat would be the hardest part, but as I just said, it's human nature to give in to old habits. Unfortunately, because food is everywhere and unhealthy foods are extremely easy to obtain (it's much easier and convenient, for example, to purchase an entire high-fat meal in a drive-through window than it is to find a restaurant offering quick, healthy, low-fat options), the temptation to fall back into old habits is ever present.

Rest assured, it does become easier to maintain good eating habits over time. The more determined you are, the better the chance that you're going to be strong enough to initiate healthy habits. The goal is to integrate those healthy routines into your daily routine or activities so that you don't even thing about them—they're just part of your new lifestyle.

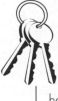

Here's to Your Heart

If you're reading this chapter thinking, "Eating low-fat foods is something that will never seem like a regular part of my day," think again. Repetition can break old habits, and determination can help you adhere to repetition. Chances are, you don't spend a lot of time thinking about the foods you eat now; they're simply part of your day. That will happen eventually with your new eating habits. Believe that you can do it, and you can make it happen.

Move It and Lose Cholesterol Points

Eating healthy foods isn't the only new routine you're going to work on! To achieve optimum health, it's important to integrate physical activity into your lifestyle, too.

Exercise is one of those sticking points with people. One bad experience can turn someone off of physical activity forever; however, finding an activity that you enjoy can make all the difference in making exercise a regular part of your day. Keep trying new activities until you find one that you actually look forward to. If you find walking boring, jazz things up with a portable CD player or iPod, or bring your dog along. Look for ways to make activity enjoyable, and eventually it won't be something you dread; it will be a normal part of your routine!

Often, people will engage in good habits (such as daily exercise) every day for many years. Over time, these habits become part of their routine, much like brushing their teeth in the morning. The key is to integrate the activity into one's routine. Over time, with consistency of participation, it becomes difficult not to engage in the activity! In fact, healthy activities over time may become effortless.

Consider the athlete who jogs every morning at 5:30. He probably wouldn't sleep in even if he could, because it would throw the rest of his morning off, 5:30 is simply his time to get up and get moving! He wasn't born running at the crack of dawn; he chose to make this part of his morning routine.

Starting Points

As I said in Chapter 7, initiating and maintaining healthy eating habits begins at the supermarket. You should purchase *only* healthy foods! Remember: after you bring it home, it's going to be eaten—and it doesn't matter what "it" is. Maybe you'll stop to buy a package of cookies that you don't even like, reasoning that they're for your spouse. When a craving for sweets and fat hits you, you may realize that you don't dislike this type of cookie nearly as much as you thought you did. We'll talk about occasionally straying from a healthy diet later in this chapter; however, it's safest to keep unhealthy foods out of the house completely.

> **Healthy Heart Facts**
>
> When you open the refrigerator, your only decision should be which healthy food to eat. This is much, much easier to do if the only foods you've brought home from the supermarket are low-fat, mostly natural options.

Similarly, healthy eating while at a restaurant involves healthy restaurant choices and healthy items on the menu. One may be able to request that food be broiled or baked or cooked in olive oil instead of butter or margarine.

The foods to avoid in a restaurant include fried foods and foods served with sauces. It's best to order food steamed, baked, broiled in its own juices, or prepared with olive oil or sunflower oil. These are all low-fat methods of preparing food.

Other tips for eating out include the following:

◆ Avoid vegetables that are cooked in sauces or in oils that are hydrogenated (such as coconut and palm oils). If there's any doubt, ask for your vegetables to be steamed or cooked in olive oil. Of course, raw vegetables are always the best.

◆ Avoid fatty meats, such as pork and lamb. It may be acceptable to have a low-fat steak, but ask for the fat to be trimmed off the meat before it's cooked.

◆ Avoid white bread. Whole-wheat bread is a better choice. If you can't abstain from the bread, at least avoid the margarine. If you have a choice between white rice and brown rice, choose the brown rice.

◆ Avoid foods high in simple sugars, such as soda. Of course, very few deserts are truly healthy except for a bowl of fresh fruit.

Being a Smart Shopper

Adapting to a low-fat diet really depends on your ability to be a smart shopper. I highly recommend following the Paleolithic diet; making the decision to eat a Paleolithic diet involves choosing appropriate foods at the supermarket, such as …

◆ **Grains and cereals.** Whole grains are best. Refined flour and white sugar are not easily digested by the body and often contribute to weight gain.

◆ **Fish.** A terrific source of omega-3 fatty acids, which has been shown to benefit the heart. Fatty fish such as salmon and tuna have the highest concentrations of fatty acids.

◆ **Lean meats.** Look for white poultry meat, such as chicken breast and turkey breast. Dark meat coming from the hind quarters (legs, thighs) is higher in fat.

◆ **Nuts.** Remember, nuts are a good source of essential fatty acids. Walnuts are especially high in omega-3 fatty acids. Watch your caloric intake here, though, as nuts have a high calorie count. (You'll recall from Chapter 7 that consuming too many calories results in extra body fat.)

◆ **Fruits and vegetables.** You can't overeat these foods, so try to get a good variety of each. Naturally, there will be some fruits and vegetables that you'll enjoy more than others.

◆ **Legumes and beans.** These are a great source of protein and are low in fat. Legumes and beans also contain chemicals called phytochemicals that may offer some protection against heart disease.

Making these foods part of your daily eating habits can only result in good health!

And what kinds of foods should you turn a blind eye to? Anything high in fat, sugar, or refined flour: Soda. Chips. Candy. Pastries. Butter. White bread. (You get the picture.) Making the right choices at the market will make it easier for you to maintain a healthy diet at home and decrease the likelihood of a relapse in a moment of weakness.

Tools to Use

A useful tool to help maintain compliance with a healthy eating regimen is an occasional deviation from the routine. Allowing yourself a weekly break can help maintain compliance in the long term with healthy eating habits.

Did you read that correctly? Did I just tell you to throw the healthy diet out the window and gorge yourself on fats and sweets? Although I don't advocate stuffing yourself with 28 bacon cheeseburgers in one sitting, an occasional dietary indiscretion can sometimes reinforce healthy eating habits later.

People tend to place too much emphasis on sticking to an extremely rigid diet plan, so much so that when an occasional slipup occurs, a person immediately feels an inordinate amount of guilt. This guilt, in turn, can lead to a destructive all-or-nothing attitude (something along the lines of, "Well, I already blew it; I might as well quit now").

Give yourself the occasional break. Oftentimes, avoidance of strict dietary compliance can have better long-term results. If you know that you can have a piece of pie for dessert when you're eating in a restaurant, for example, you're less likely to feel the pressure of avoiding treats all the time. The key is to see these food items as occasional indulgences, and not as everyday staples in your diet.

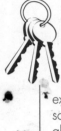

> ### Here's to Your Heart
>
> It's all right to indulge yourself once in a while, but don't set yourself up for a downward spiral into consistent bad habits. If you choose to have a treat at home, purchase one small serving (a single slice of cake, for example, or a one-ounce bag of chips). Treating yourself in a restaurant is often a safe option because you won't have the extra servings in your home. If you're a guest in someone else's home, try to resist the social obligation to indulge in high-fat treats (here's your chance to educate your friends about the Paleolithic diet!), or request a tiny piece of cake or pie.

Sample Menus

Purchasing the raw materials for a healthy diet is a great start. Knowing how to assemble them at mealtimes is the next logical step. This section includes some sample menus of healthy Paleolithic diets.

Breakfast

You know breakfast is the most important meal of the day, but it's hard to get going when you're weighed down with bacon and sausage. These are healthy breakfast items that you can eat in any combination:

◆ Coffee, without sugar, with a nondairy creamer; bottled water; carbonated diet soda; fruit juice with no added sugar; skim or nonfat milk.

◆ Bananas, apples, pears, grapes, plums, nectarines, grapefruit, oranges, apricots, melons (including watermelon or cantaloupe).

◆ A mixture of various nuts consisting of peanuts, cashews, seeds, pecans and walnuts. About ½ cup every day is best.

◆ One bowlful of granola without added sugar.

♦ Two to three hard-boiled eggs twice a week.

♦ One can of tuna fish in water with low-fat mayonnaise. One to two tablespoons of low-fat mayo should be enough to make the tuna tasty.

Lunch

When lunch time rolls around, don't toss your request into the office take-out order. Instead, pack your own lunch in the morning. It can include:

♦ Follow the previous recommendations for breakfast beverages.

♦ Can of tuna fish with or without low-fat, low calorie mayonnaise.

♦ A tossed green salad consisting of lettuce, tomatoes, cucumbers, green peppers, sprouts, and mushrooms. Top with lemon juice, vinegar, and olive oil or any other oil that is mono- or polyunsaturated.

♦ Vegetables: eggplant, potatoes, sweet potatoes, corn, carrots, celery, broccoli, cauliflower, and peas. In general, a bowl of vegetables should be adequate. The American Heart Association recommends seven servings per day, so the more, the better!

♦ Legumes: beans of all types, lentils. A bowl is sufficient, but again, the more, the better.

Dinner

Dinnertime is not synonymous with drive-thru fare! Healthy eating doesn't mean that it's tasteless or boring. There are many options available for low-fat dinners, including:

♦ Again, follow recommendations for beverages listed in the Breakfast section.

♦ Salmon, trout, halibut, or other fish broiled, steamed, or cooked in canola, sunflower, safflower, or olive oil.

A six-ounce serving of salmon or other fatty fish is adequate. Of course, there is no harm to eating more than six ounces of fish. The amount of oil added should be minimized. If you're preparing your own fish, ¼ cup should be adequate oil for cooking. The most important factor is to minimize oil consumption. Most oils will raise cholesterol and LDL. The importance of cooking with a less-saturated oils is that you're making a choice of substituting an unsaturated oil for a saturated one.

- Boiled or broiled poultry, skinless.

- Tossed salad, as above for lunch.

- Vegetables as listed above for lunch.

- For dessert, try some of the fresh fruits listed above for breakfast.

- Red meat is acceptable once a week.

- It is acceptable to deviate from the diet once a week.

- If dressing on your salad is a must, look for one that's low-fat and low-sugar (and low-calorie).

Sometimes it makes sense to ingest a few calories and a small amount of fat to allow the salad to be palatable. In general, though, I would suggest trying to avoid bottled dressings because there may be hidden calories, including sugar calories. Oil, vinegar and lemon juice are good alternatives.

A slice of bread or two can be added to a meal. Good breads include Ezekiel breads and whole wheat breads. Multigrain breads are also good. The importance is to consume bread not made with white flour, which is devoid of nutritive value. If you have a choice between using margarine, butter, or olive oil on your bread, choose the olive oil.

The Least You Need to Know

- Cholesterol reduction depends on a three-pronged approach including diet, exercise, and appropriate medications.

- Maintaining a healthy lifestyle requires dedication and vigilance.

- Learning to view exercise as a normal part of your day will make it easier for you to stick with it.

- Healthy eating begins in the supermarket; leave unhealthy foods there!

- Giving yourself the occasional break from a healthy diet might just increase your chances of staying with it in the long term.

Part 3

Mind and Body Approaches for Lowering Cholesterol

Exercise is a great way to lower "bad" cholesterol and raise "good" cholesterol. So in Part 3, we also take a look at how to ease into a lifestyle that includes regular physical activity. But don't worry! This doesn't involve signing yourself up for a triathlon or even joining a gym. It's easy to work more activity into your day if you start thinking that *every little bit helps* (as opposed to thinking that you just aren't up to the task of running a mini-marathon, so there's no sense in getting off the couch). Part 3 teaches you plenty of things that you didn't know the mind and body were capable of doing for heart-health. And the best part is that *you* are in control!

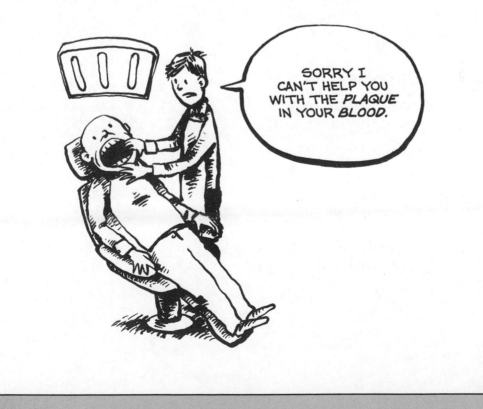

SORRY I CAN'T HELP YOU WITH THE *PLAQUE* IN YOUR *BLOOD*.

Chapter 14

Getting Fit

In This Chapter

- Learn the guidelines to know how much heart-healthy activity you need each week
- Understand why exercise benefits your body and mind
- Convince yourself that you do not need to run a marathon to become fit
- Read about heart failure and exercise intolerance
- Discover the truth about being fat and fit

Typically to get fit, you must start an exercise program that involves low-level physical activity that you can tolerate well. Common sense dictates that if you're struggling to make it through an exercise or activity, you're probably not going to be motivated to do it again; for this reason, doctors advise starting slowly and gradually increasing activity. It is unnecessary to become an athlete or engage in high-intensity or strenuous physical activity to gain health benefits from exercise.

Many studies have been performed over the years to determine the optimum amount of physical activity necessary to enjoy good health. It turns out that most of the beneficial effects from exercise on cardiac health are achieved with moderate exercise. In this chapter, we'll talk about your current physical condition and how this impacts your ability to become more physically fit.

Assessing Your Current Physical Condition

The key element to exercise is to start slow and increase your exercise level gradually. This concept of "start slow, go slow" is partly derived from cardiac rehabilitation programs, which are exercise programs for patients who have had heart attacks, coronary-artery bypass surgery, or heart failure. Many patients in these programs are elderly with other medical conditions that limit their exercise abilities; a good percentage of them haven't exercised for many years and have fears and anxieties surrounding starting an exercise program in the context of known heart disease.

Healthy Heart Facts
The American Heart Association has determined that approximately 20 to 30 minutes of exercise per day, 5 to 7 days per week, is a level of activity sufficient to achieve the health benefits of exercise.

If elderly men and women who are unfamiliar with exercise and who have cardiac conditions that limit their exercise level can start a program of cardiac rehabilitation and achieve health benefits, you can, too! In relation to elderly heart patients, it's easier for younger people to either start a program or increase their level of activity.

Healthy Heart Facts
The key concept to begin an exercise program is to increase your activity level and then continue to remain active and exercise over the long term. Just like making healthy food choices, exercise entails consistent vigilance and willpower. Over time, regular exercise becomes part of your normal routine and thus easier to maintain.

Exercise and Cholesterol

Getting fit by engaging in an exercise program has been shown in various studies to decrease LDL, triglycerides, and total cholesterol. Exercise also increases HDL. The greatest benefits are achieved when exercise and diet are combined with medication (when appropriate). Consistent, daily exercise has the greatest advantages for heart health.

Exercise does not need to be high intensity to be beneficial. Actually, the greatest benefits are achieved by simply starting to exercise (in other words, getting off the couch). Exercise that increases the heart rate and achieves cardiovascular benefit is best. These activities improve aerobic conditioning and fitness and decrease cholesterol.

Slow and Steady Wins the Race

When you decide to start an exercise program, your baseline level of fitness is not that important. What's more important is to achieve a change in your current activity level. *Activity should be increased.* This is the important point. Whatever your baseline level of exercise participation, you should strive to do more.

Relatively healthy people with elevated cholesterol should not necessarily seek to become elite athletes. Sudden, intense exercising may not be beneficial for several reasons: first, dramatic changes in your activity or exercise level may increase your risk for injury. Injuries, in turn, often dissuade people from resuming exercise after the injury heals. In addition, it's difficult to continue an intense exercise program that has been started overnight. The gradual integration of exercise into your daily routine makes it more likely that you'll continue on with it and less likely that you'll return to your old, inactive ways.

def•i•ni•tion

Physical fitness is really a term that describes how much exercise a person can tolerate.

Healthy Heart Facts
Studies that have looked at cholesterol reduction using diet alone versus using diet plus exercise revealed that the greatest benefits were achieved when aerobic exercise was added to a heart-healthy diet.

What's Your Level?

There are some fairly sophisticated ways of measuring how much oxygen your heart extracts from the blood during exercise. These methods are a reflection of how much oxygen is delivered to the heart with activity or exercise level. As exercise intensity increases, the heart's oxygen requirements and delivery increase. A healthy heart and cardiovascular system can increase delivery of oxygen consistent with the heart's requirements. However, people who have physical conditions limiting their heart's abilities to utilize oxygen or deliver the necessary oxygen to the heart may not be able to work at higher exercise levels.

For example, a person who has had several heart attacks because of a sudden blood clot in an artery and who has experienced heart muscle loss due to this sudden occlusion of blood flow may have difficulty delivering adequate blood to the heart during exercise. This person is likely to become short of breath while exercising.

Exercise and the Condition of Your Heart

The problem of difficulty in delivering adequate blood flow to the exercising muscles due to a problem with the heart and circulation is called *heart failure*. There are many definitions of heart failure; however, one thing that all individuals with heart failure have in common is decreased exercise tolerance.

def•i•ni•tion

Heart failure is a term used to describe the inability of the heart and blood vessels to provide adequate blood flow, nutrients, and oxygen to the rest of the body.

You don't need to suffer a heart attack to have heart failure. Many of the risk factors that have been discussed in this book—such as high blood pressure, diabetes, and obesity—can lead to heart failure. Often, a doctor will see a patient who has several risk factors for heart disease and is complaining of symptoms of diminishing exercise tolerance and shortness of breath, but who hasn't had a heart attack. This person may be suffering from heart failure without ever having had a heart attack.

Classifying Heart Failure and Exercise Tolerance

There are two classifications of heart failure; these are important because they help to determine a heart failure patient's level of exercise fitness. We'll discuss one method of classifying heart failure in this section, and the other in the following section.

The first classification has been around for a long time and is referred to as the *New York Heart Association Classification*, which has four categories:

The Doctor Says

Other symptoms of heart failure include swelling of the legs, increased urination, fatigue, or shortness of breath while lying flat.

- **Category I** is normal exercise tolerance, with no limitation.

- **Category II** is shortness of breath, exercise limitation, or difficulty with ordinary activity.

- **Category III** is shortness of breath, exercise intolerance, or difficulty with less than ordinary activity.

- **Category IV** is shortness of breath, difficulty with exercise, or difficulty at rest.

Overall, about half of the people diagnosed with heart disease die within five years. Some studies show an even higher mortality. People who have heart failure and exercise limitation have a median survival of one to three years. We can clearly see that the exercise intolerance characteristic of heart failure (that is, the degree to which a patient is unable to tolerate physical activity) is highly lethal.

The Doctor Says

Many more people are afflicted with heart failure than with cancer in the United States, and a diagnosis of heart failure has a higher mortality than advanced cancer. In addition, the degree of exercise intolerance correlates linearly with mortality—this means that individuals who have the worst exercise tolerance have the highest mortality.

Staging Heart Failure and Exercise Intolerance

Another way that doctors classify heart failure and exercise intolerance is by stages: A and B.

Stage A heart failure is a situation where a person feels well and can exercise, but has significant risk factors. An example would be a man with high blood pressure who feels just fine. This person is at risk for developing heart failure with symptoms of exercise intolerance.

People with *Stage B heart failure* still have the risk factors that those with Stage A have. However, Stage B involves a weakened heart muscle—as a result, these people have more exercise intolerance. Usually, these people have no symptoms at all with ordinary activity, but may develop shortness of breath at increasing exercise loads.

Stages C and D heart failure are progressive degrees of exercise intolerance and heart muscle weakness ultimately leading to death. All four stages can be treated with medications.

"Before Beginning Any Exercise Program ..."

You've heard the warnings on exercise tapes and DVDs. Don't begin an exercise program without first checking with your doctor, especially if you have risk factors for cardiovascular disease!

People with heart failure are clearly physically unfit and should see their physician before starting an exercise program. If you have the risk factors that are discussed in this book, it's possible that you may have exercise intolerance and be physically unfit. If you have these risk factors, you should see your physician before you start an exercise program. Your physician may need to stabilize your health first. The good news is that even individuals with heart failure—even quite advanced heart failure—will benefit from exercise and become physically more fit.

The Doctor Says

Heart arteries that are narrowed by cholesterol deposits are sensitive to chemicals and hormones in the blood that cause the blood vessels to constrict. Obviously, an already narrowed artery doesn't need anything narrowing it even further. If this is a concern, your doctor can do a test to assess the effects of stress on the heart (called a *stress test*) and to evaluate your response to physical activity.

Let's say you have several risk factors for heart disease, but no symptoms and no recent changes in your exercise tolerance. You're likely to be fit enough to undergo an exercise program; however, anyone who has any doubt about their ability to start a program should see their doctor first. Moreover, it is a good idea for to visit your physician even if you only have risk factors, as often the level of risk is greater than you might estimate.

Assuming that you do not have exercise limitation and you got the go-ahead from your physician that exercise is safe, it's time to get fit. In the next chapter, we talk about devising an exercise program.

Fat and Fit Versus Lean and Unfit

Americans focus on weight loss for its cosmetic and aesthetic effects. Weight loss and avoidance of obesity (those aesthetic effects I'm talking about) necessitate a two-pronged approach to weight loss: diet and exercise. Fortunately, the positive effects of exercise carry over to the heart no matter how much weight loss is involved.

Benefits of a Two-Pronged Approach

People who lose weight by beginning an exercise program and adopting a healthy diet experience greater health benefits than if they lose weight by dieting alone. Studies indicate that overweight people who exercise on a regular basis and who become physically fit become healthier—and they don't have to become stick-thin to achieve health benefits. So, in other words, if you have a choice between being fat and physically fit or being lean and unfit, it's better to be overweight and physically fit.

Now, read that paragraph again. It doesn't say that it's best to be obese, or that being overweight is ideal. It says that anyone who gets involved in a physical fitness program is going to reap some health benefits from it, and that getting up off the couch is far better for your health than doing nothing, even if you happen to be thin already. Getting that heart pumping on a regular basis (and with your doctor's approval) is the key to good health, no matter what your size.

> **Healthy Heart Facts**
>
> To diet and exercise for health benefits, the goal should be to combine daily exercise with a healthy Paleolithic diet that reduces cholesterol.

Here's to Your Heart

If fat and fit is better than lean and unfit, it stands to reason that lean and fit must be the most beneficial to the heart and body!

Exercise is a necessary component of any health program. It reduces cholesterol and improves the health of the heart. The studies in medical literature which have demonstrated a reduction in cardiovascular mortality with medication have also shown a reduction in cardiac events (such as heart attack) with diet and exercise, especially when medication was also used.

Exercise Really Does Feel Good

The reason why becoming active and physically fit is so important is that exercise has a significant protective effect against many diseases. And in addition to its pleasing physical effects (such as weight loss), exercise has a powerful anti-depressant and mood-enhancing effect. So if you've noticed that you feel lousy before you take a walk and that you feel uplifted afterwards, you're not imagining things! The positive effect of exercise on mood and outlook even helps to improve a person's ability to deal with a chronic problem, such as elevated cholesterol or even heart failure.

Here's to Your Heart

Exercise is important for mental health. A major component to maintaining an exercise program and taking medications on a daily basis is a positive outlook, daily vigilance, and conscientiousness. Exercise can help to lift your mood, improve your attitude, and make you feel physically well.

Many of the ways by which exercise improves physical and mental well-being are not completely understood. However, we know that people who have heart failure and who exercise develop an adaptation at the level of their muscles to the poor circulation that is intrinsic to the heart failure problem. In other words, when the heart is failing to deliver adequate circulation to the body, the muscles attempt to compensate. Exercising muscle develops certain biochemical changes that allow it to extract more oxygen, even from poor circulation.

And again, if people who are ill with heart failure can benefit from exercise, a relatively healthy person who has risk factors for heart disease later in life (such as high blood pressure, obesity and diabetes) can certainly reap these benefits also.

The Least You Need to Know

- One should exercise approximately 30 minutes per day 5 to 7 days per week.

- Some individuals will have long-standing heart disease risk factors that may put them at risk for heart failure.

- Some individuals may already have early heart failure as an explanation for their reduced exercise tolerance and exercise limitation.

- When someone decides to commence an exercise program, his or her baseline level of fitness is less important.

- Working exercise into your daily routine gradually will help you to keep at it in the long run.

Chapter 15

Building an Exercise Program

In This Chapter

- ◆ Evaluate your own fitness level
- ◆ Learn the difference between isometric and isotonic exercises
- ◆ See sample workouts for every level of fitness
- ◆ Gain insight into training with weights safely
- ◆ Know why you need to talk to your doctor before starting an exercise program

When you build an exercise program for yourself, you need to work your exercise goals, age, conditioning, and any associated illnesses into the plan. Healthy people that are interested in lowering their cholesterol and improving their fitness level can begin a program after talking with a doctor. Some people may be referred to an exercise physiologist, a physical trainer, or even a physician who has expertise and experience with *exercise prescription*, detailing which exercises may be ideal for their age and physical condition.

Activity should be increased gradually as exercise tolerance improves and, ideally, an exercise program should be maintained for life…so it's as important to find the right type of exercise for yourself as it is to get up and get moving! This chapter includes sample exercises that are good for anyone at any age and any level of fitness.

Finding an Exercise Plan That Works for You

In theory, at least, exercise comes in two basic varieties: *isometric*, which is resistance training, and *isotonic*, which involves aerobic and cardiovascular conditioning. In reality, though, pure isometric and pure isotonic exercises don't exist. All exercise is a combination of isometric and isotonic exercise. For example, although weightlifting is primarily isometric, there's also an isotonic component to it. People who want to achieve *aerobic* benefit from weightlifting can increase the number of repetitions or frequency of lifts and perform the exercise routine rapidly to increase their heart rate. Similarly, bicycling, although primarily an isometric exercise, yields isometric benefits because while it gets the heart pumping, it also conditions muscles in the process.

Most programs can be tailored to the goals of the individual. Exercise programs should also be customized to your level of exercise conditioning, age, and any underlying injuries or illnesses.

def•i•ni•tion

> Your doctor can provide you with an **exercise prescription,** which is detailed advice regarding how much and what type of physical activity is appropriate for you.
>
> **Isometric exercise** refers to resistance training, or using a weight or load to condition muscles.
>
> **Isotonic exercise** refers to **aerobic conditioning,** or strengthening the heart and cardiovascular system.

Isometrics

Isometric exercise is resistance training, a form of exercise in which an individual works a muscle or group of muscles against a resistance load, such as a weight. The weight may be a free weight, such as a barbell or dumbbell, or it might be a machine, such as a Nautilus or Universal exercise machine. Resistance training may also involve carrying heavy objects, wrestling, or performing exercises against your own weight (such as doing push-ups, sit-ups, or pull-ups).

Isometric exercise increases muscle strength, power, and size. A bodybuilder, football player, wrestler, or boxer might be interested in developing strength and muscle size. Power-lifters and bodybuilders are extreme examples of people who have relied on weight training to achieve their exercise goals. When performed rapidly enough, weight training can yield cardiovascular or aerobic benefits in addition to increasing muscle strength and size.

Isotonics

Isotonic exercise is aerobic training; this kind of activity doesn't use a weight load to strengthen muscles, but rather you exercises muscles in such a way that achieves aerobic and cardiovascular benefits. Examples of isotonic exercise include the following activities:

◆ Swimming

◆ Jogging

◆ Walking

◆ Jumping rope

◆ Bicycling

> **Healthy Heart Facts**
>
> Any exercise program consists of three basic components: warm-up, exercise, and cool-down. Whatever form of exercise you choose, take care to include these components every time you exercise to avoid injury. You'll maximize your safety and also encourage your own long-term participation in the activity.

This list provides a better example of how all exercises are combinations of isometric and isotonic. Each exercise on this list strengthens both the heart and the muscles. For example, if you're not a runner and you go for a run anyway, you'll feel your heart and your leg muscles are working overtime!

A Level Playing Field

For simplicity, we'll break all exercise programs down into three levels, which are based on the baseline condition of each individual: low, medium, and high.

Exercise level is relative to the physical condition of the person performing the exercise! This is important to keep in mind, as anyone beginning an exercise program should progress from low to medium to high over time. A 17-year-old high-school football player may view a four-hour practice as low-level exercise, for example, whereas a 75-year-old male who has led a sedentary lifestyle may view a 30-minute walk to work as a high-level activity. So, because people vary according to their baseline level of exercise conditioning, we can further divide them into three distinct groups: low fitness level, medium fitness level, and high fitness level. (Our 17-year-old football player would be characterized as functioning at a high fitness level, of course, while we would say our elderly male was functioning at a low fitness level.)

It's important that the elderly male not try to work up to the level of the football player, for several reasons, the most obvious of which is that his heart and body are not conditioned well enough to withstand that level of activity. Each individual has to fairly evaluate herself and work at the level that suits her physical conditioning at the time. There's no sense to make yourself feel like a failure because you can't run a marathon right now. Find an exercise that will benefit your health, and you'll eventually work up to a higher level.

Choose Your Level

To develop an exercise plan, you should classify yourself within one of the three fitness levels and start with a low-level program, eventually working toward a high-level program. Ideally, you should spend about three to six months at each level and increase activity somewhat within each level over several weeks. This section will list some sample programs to choose from.

Low Fitness Level/Low Level Exercise:

Walking on level surface for 10 minutes per day, 5 to 7 days per week, gradually increasing to 20 minutes per day

Swimming 1 to 2 laps at slow pace, gradually increasing to 3 to 4 laps, 5 to 7 days per week

Bicycling over level surface at slow pace for 10 minutes per day, gradually increasing to 20 minutes per day, 5 to 7 days per week

Low Fitness Level/Moderate Level Exercise:

Slow-pace walking over level surface for 30 minutes per day

Swimming at slow pace 4 to 5 laps per day, 5 to 7 days per week

Bicycling over level surface at a slow pace up to 30 minutes per day

Jumping rope 1 minute, 3 times (with a 2-minute rest between sets)

Low Fitness Level/High Level Exercise:

Moderate-pace walking over level surface for 30 minutes per day, 5 to 7 days per week

Swimming 5 to 10 laps per day at a slow pace, 5 to 7 days per week

Bicycling over level surface at a slow pace up to 30 minutes per day at a rapid pace, 5 to 7 days per week

Jumping rope $1\frac{1}{2}$ minutes $\times$ 3 (2 minutes rest in between sets)

Moderate Fitness Level/Low Level Exercise:

Walking on level surface at moderate pace for 30 minutes per day, incorporating 1 incline comprising up to 10 percent of the trip, 5 to 7 days per week

Swimming 5 to 10 laps per day at a moderate pace, 5 to 7 days per week

Bicycling over level surface at a moderate pace up to 30 minutes per day, riding up at least 1 incline that makes up about 10 percent of the trip, 5 to 7 days per week

Moderate Fitness Level/Moderate Level Exercise:

Walking on level surface at moderate pace for 30 minutes per day, incorporating 2 inclines that comprise up to 20 percent of the trip, 5 to 7 days per week.

Swimming 10 to 15 laps per day at a moderate pace, 5 to 7 days per week.

Bicycling over level surface at a moderate rate up to 30 minutes per day, incorporating 2 inclines comprising up to 20 percent of the trip, 5 to 7 days per week.

Jumping rope 1½ minutes × 3 (1-minute rest in between sets).

Moderate Fitness Level/High Level Exercise:

Walking on level surface at moderate pace for 30 minutes per day, incorporating 3 inclines comprising up to 30 percent of the trip, 5 to 7 days per week.

Swimming 15 to 20 laps per day at a moderate pace, 5 to 7 days per week.

Bicycling over level surface at a moderate pace up to 30 minutes per day, incorporating 3 inclines comprising up to 30 percent of the trip, 5 to 7 days per week.

Jumping rope 1½ minutes × 3 (30-second rest between sets).

High Fitness Level/Low Level Exercise:

Walking 30 minutes per day at rapid pace, incorporating up to 3 inclines comprising up to 30 percent of the trip, 5 to 7 days per week.

Swimming 15 to 20 laps per day at a rapid pace, 5 to 7 days per week.

Bicycling over level surface at a rapid pace up to 30 minutes per day, incorporating 3 inclines comprising up to 30 percent of the trip, 5 to 7 days per week.

High Fitness Level/Moderate Level Exercise:

Walking 30 minutes per day at rapid pace, incorporating up to 4 inclines, comprising up to 40 percent of the trip, 5 to 7 days per week.

Swimming 20 to 25 laps per day at a rapid pace, 5 to 7 days per week.

Bicycling over level surface at a rapid pace up to 30 minutes per day, incorporating 4 inclines comprising up to 40 percent of the trip, 5 to 7 days per week.

Jumping rope 2 minutes × 3 (1-minute rest between sets).

High Fitness Level/High Level Exercise:

Walking 30 minutes per day at rapid pace, incorporating up to 5 inclines, comprising up to 50 percent of the trip, 5 to 7 days per week.

Swimming 25 to 30 laps per day at a rapid pace, 5 to 7 days per week.

Bicycling over level surface at a rapid pace up to 30 minutes per day, incorporating up to 5 inclines comprising up to 50 percent of the trip, 5 to 7 days per week.

Jumping rope 2 minutes × 3 (30-second rest).

Resistance Training/Weight Training

The following program can be used for strength training or building muscle size and bulk. Weight training is performed as sets of repetitions. Each movement is a *repetition*. A series of repetition is called a *set*. You should work out with weights for 3 to 6 months before expecting to see results. People at all levels of fitness and at all levels of exercise tolerance can utilize weight training.

Beginners: First 6 month

Upper Body: 3 days per week

- Bench press: 3 sets × 10 to 12 reps
- Military press: 3 sets × 10 to 12 reps
- Barbell curls or dumbbell curls: 3 sets × 10 to 12 reps
- Triceps overhead presses: 3 sets × 10 to 12 reps
- Seated latissimus dorsi pull-downs: 3 sets × 1 to 12 reps

Lower body: 3 days per week

- ◆ Squats or deep knee bends: 3 sets × 10 to 12 reps

- ◆ Leg extensions: 3 sets × 1 to 12 reps

- ◆ Leg curls: 3 sets × 10 to 12 reps

- ◆ Standing calf raises: 3 sets × 10 to 12 reps

- ◆ Sit-ups: 6 days per week; 3 sets × 15 reps

Intermediate: 6 months to 1 year

Upper body: 2 days per week

- ◆ Bench press: 4 sets × 6 to 8 reps

- ◆ Military press: 4 sets × 6 to 8 reps

- ◆ Triceps bench press: 4 sets × 6 to 8 reps

- ◆ Seated latissimus dorsi pull-downs: 4 sets × 6 to 8 reps

- ◆ Seated rows: 4 sets × 6 to 8 reps

- ◆ Barbell curls or dumbbell curls: 4 sets × 6 to 8 reps

- ◆ Pull-ups: 3 sets × 5 to 8 reps

- ◆ Dips: 3 sets × 5 to 8 reps

- ◆ Wrist curls: 3 sets × 6 to 8 reps

Lower Body

- ◆ Squats or deep knee bends: 4 sets of 6 to 8 reps

- ◆ Leg extensions: 4 sets of 6 to 8 reps

- ◆ Leg curls: 4 sets of 6 to 8 reps

- ◆ Standing calf curls: 4 sets of 6 to 8 reps

- ◆ Sit-ups: 6 days per week; 3 sets of 25 reps

Advanced: 1 to 2 years

Upper Body: 2 days per week

- ◆ Bench press: 5 sets × 3 to 5 reps

- Incline bench press: 5 sets × 3 to 5 reps

- Triceps bench press: 5 sets × 3 to 5 reps

- Military presses: 5 sets × 3 to 5 reps

- Barbell curls: 5 sets × 3 to 5 reps

- Reverse barbell curls: 5 sets 3 to 5 reps

- Bent over barbell rows with variable grip: 5 sets × 3 to 5 reps

- Triceps presses overhead: 5 sets × 3 to 5 reps

- Seated pull-downs: 5 sets × 3 to 5 reps

- Seated rows: 5 sets × 3 to 5 reps

- Dips, weighted: 5 sets × 3 to 5 reps

- Pull-ups, weighted: 5 sets × 3 to 5 reps

- Wrist curls: 5 sets × 3 to 5 reps

Lower Body: 2 days per week

- Squats or deep knee bends: 5 sets × 3 to 5 reps

- Leg extensions: 5 sets × 3 to 5 reps

- Leg curls: 5 sets × 3 to 5 reps

- Standing calf raises: 5 sets × 3 to 5 reps

- Sit-ups: 3 sets × 50 reps

Basic Concepts of Weight Training

As you gain strength working with weights, you should slowly add weight in 1-pound, 2½-pound, and 5-pound increments, as tolerated. For maximum strength, strive to use as much weight as possible; however, always train with a partner or a trainer for safety (and for encouragement).

Certain exercises such as bench presses should only be performed with a partner, called a spotter. A spotter should be able to help with the lift, so that you can continue to exercise to the point of exhaustion. Ideally, a trainer is required for maximum gains. One or two spotters should be present for squats. Squatting should only be performed in a rack. A rack can catch the weight if the lifter cannot lift the weight.

Weight lifting requires excruciating attention to physical form. Weightlifting with poor form puts you at high risk for injury and wastes your time to boot, as you'll only see results from using proper form. In addition, weightlifting can be physically demanding during the exercise itself and requires proper breathing technique. Exercised muscles are likely to be sore the following day or two. Soreness is a good sign, as it implies a good workout. Avoid working the same body parts on two consecutive days, and get lots of sleep and proper nutrition for best results.

Working With Your Doctor

Before beginning an exercise program, you should inform your doctor about your intent. (And if you don't have a doctor, find one. It's that important.) Your doctor needs to examine you and rule out underlying (and possible asymptomatic) heart disease.

If you have high cholesterol, it's possible that you already have heart disease. This should be treated while you're starting an exercise program. In addition, someone with elevated cholesterol is likely to have other risk factors for heart disease. (You'll remember from Chapter 5 that risk factors tend to cluster together). Individuals with clusters of risk factors are more likely to have heart disease.

The good news, of course, is that exercise is likely to be beneficial not only for elevated cholesterol but also for the cluster of risk factors. However, if you develop any new symptoms during exercise, you should immediately inform your doctor. Symptoms of chest discomfort, new shortness of breath, or palpitations are particularly worrisome.

The Doctor Says

There are certain heart muscle and electrical disorders that may develop at a young age and increase a person's risk of adverse health effects when participating in exercise. Preathletic screening helps to diagnose these individuals early.

Some people shouldn't participate in any moderate or high-intensity exercises at all. A doctor can determine whether you need an electrocardiogram, exercise treadmill, stress test, or echocardiogram before beginning an exercise program.

The Least You Need to Know

◆ You should develop an exercise program that is customized to your own level of exercise tolerance and fitness.

◆ An exercise program should start slowly and increase in activity over time for maximum health benefits.

◆ The most important component to an exercise program is that you stick with it.

◆ After you learn how to exercise and how your body responds to activity, you can modify your program, adding new components and new challenges to keep things interesting.

Chapter 16

Meditation

In This Chapter

- ◆ Understand the connection between the mind and your health
- ◆ Learn about the balance between the sympathetic and parasympathetic nervous system
- ◆ Find out how chronic stress affects your health
- ◆ Close your eyes and give meditation a try!

Our bodies and our minds are connected in a way that we most often fail to acknowledge. We live day-to-day knowing how we feel physically and mentally, but somehow, we never stop to think how one affects the other, or that there's any kind of link between the two states of being. How wrong we are!

Heart attacks are often preceded by emotional arguments with spouses and loved ones. An anxious state of mind can disrupt a plaque, leading to its rupture and subsequent blood clot that ends in a heart attack. We also know that anger and hostility, when viewed as general personality traits, are associated with an increased risk for heart attack and sudden death. Depression takes its toll, too: post–heart attack depression is associated with an increased risk of death. Socially isolated individuals have an increased risk of dying after a heart attack.

So what's to be done? We don't have a happy pill that can clear up anxiety and sadness in the mind; however, training the mind to focus and relax can have powerful health benefits. In this chapter, we'll talk what stress does to the body first; then we'll talk about meditation as a means of encouraging emotional and physical well-being.

Why It Works

A stress test is done by a cardiologist to help risk stratify or confirm a pretest decision he has made that there is a good chance that there could be a blockage in one or more blood vessels within the heart.

The Doctor Says

Although excess stress can have an adverse effect on the heart, stress reduction techniques, such as meditation, can improve blood vessel and heart health.

Similarly, a *mental stress test* is sometimes performed to determine the effect of mental stress on the heart. Instead of being instructed to exercise, the person is attached to an electrocardiogram and asked to perform mental arithmetic under conditions of increasing stress and complexity. Changes are frequently seen on the electrocardiograms of people who have cholesterol deposits and plaque in their arteries; these people will also often exhibit symptoms of chest discomfort during these stressful mental activities!

The mental stress test demonstrates how powerful an effect the mind has on the heart and blood vessels. The mind is so powerful that it can actually trigger a heart attack with an adequate amount of stress!

def•i•ni•tion

A **stress test** may be done by a cardiologist to evaluate the effect of physical or mental stress on the heart. The latter test is called a **mental stress test;** it measures how a person's heart responds to situations of increasing emotional stress and can predict the likelihood of a person developing a heart attack or stroke under similar emotional circumstances.

Fight or Flight

Our thoughts, anxieties, and fears can affect the health of our hearts and blood vessels. There is a large body of medical literature that links the presence or absence of acute and chronic stress, obsessive disorders, depression, and hostility with an increased risk for heart attack, stroke, sudden cardiac death, and hypertension. Likewise, there are also studies linking spiritual attitudes such as faith, positive thinking, and hope, as well as the presence of social support systems and a connection with community, with decreased mortality due to cardiovascular diseases.

The link between these behaviors and cardio-vascular disease may be due to our genetically programmed *fight-or-flight* response. Millions of years ago, humans developed protective adaptive mechanisms to protect themselves against impending threats. The classic example of the caveman and the sabertooth tiger illustrates this point. The caveman confronted with this kind of threat would experience a surge in adrenaline, which served to energize the caveman to deal with the threat.

def•i•ni•tion

When you feel threatened, the sympathetic nervous system kicks in and initiates a **fight-or-flight** response, fueled by adrenaline. In the short term, this is a protective measure, but if you're stressed all the time, it can be harmful to your health.

We recognize similar threats in our daily lives, and our response is close to what it would have been millions of years ago. For example, when someone walks down a dark alley and hears footsteps, the fright of this potential danger causes the body to release adrenaline. Many organs and organ systems are able to respond to this surge in adrenaline. For example, when we feel threatened …

- The pupils become dilated in order to allow us to better spot the attacker.
- The heart races and beats stronger to provide more blood to the body.
- The blood vessels in the skin constrict to move blood away from the skin in case there is bleeding.

Another example of the fight-or-flight response are the stories of superhuman strength during situations of extreme danger.

Chronic Anxiety and the Heart

The heart is one organ that's highly responsive to adrenaline. When someone experiences a heart attack, adrenaline and similar compounds are released in the body. These compounds allow the heart to muster reserve strength to better the person's chances of survival. However, over time, the activation of the adrenaline system can cause the heart to fail by depleting it of energy. Suffice it to say that the heart and other organs experience a detrimental effect over time when there is persistent or chronic activation of the adrenaline system.

The adrenaline system is also called the *sympathetic nervous system*, which makes the body work harder. The opposite of the sympathetic nervous system is the *parasympathetic nervous system*, which slows things down by relaxing the heart and other organs. The sympathetic nervous system is meant for acute responses to threats. Chronic states of sympathetic nervous system activation are not good for the body.

def•i•ni•tion

The body's autonomic (or involuntary) systems are controlled by the **sympathetic nervous system,** which makes organs work harder, and the **parasympathetic nervous system,** which has a more relaxing effect on the body.

Normally, the parasympathetic system is the dominant force in the body's state of balance. When there's an imbalance between sympathetic and parasympathetic nervous systems such that the sympathetic nervous system prevails over time, the heart and other organs may fail.

Chronic anxiety and stress can, theoretically, lead to chronic activation of the sympathetic nervous system and the illnesses that follow, such as heart attack and stroke. Sympathetic nervous system activity increases the likelihood of plaque rupture and heart attack because it activates inflammatory cells in the body. This in turn makes the platelets more sticky so that they are more likely to clump together and cause heart attacks and strokes.

Although it's never been shown definitively that chronic stress increases risk for heart attack and stroke, there's a solid database linking it to heart disease. Consequently, it's not hard to also form a hypothesis that relaxation techniques and interventions that reduce anxiety may reduce risk for heart attack, stroke, sudden death, and hypertension.

Placebos and the Mind

For those whose question the plausibility of the mind-body connection, consider the magnitude and power of the *placebo effect*. It has been demonstrated many times that interventions that are believed to improve health or relief pain and suffering may actually be effective based upon an individual's belief that they will work.

An example of the placebo effect is one particular treatment for *angina*, which is chest pain due to blockages in their arteries. Angina is typically relieved with medication, angioplasty (you'll recall we talked about this procedure in Chapter 6), and bypass surgery. Some patients have angina that is not relieved even after several different therapies have been tried.

In recent years, a technique called *transmyocardial laser revascularization* has been used to treat stubborn angina pain. In theory, this allows blood and oxygen to percolate through the muscle. However, in reality, this is not likely to be the mechanism of pain relief. It's believed that the often-dramatic benefits experienced by patients are due to the *placebo effect*, a form of pain relief or therapy that works because of the patient's belief that it is going to work! The placebo effect demonstrates the power that the mind has over our physical well-being.

def•i•ni•tion

The **placebo effect** refers to the belief that a certain therapy has worked because we thought that it would, despite evidence suggesting that the therapy did not work.

Another classic example of the placebo effect are the clinical studies in which one group of subjects are given medication for headache or pain and another group is given sugar pills or pills containing some other inert ingredient. Neither group knows whether they've been given the real medication. Time and time again, patients who have received the sugar pills have reported relief of their pain. Because they believe the medication *should* work, it *does* work.

The placebo effect lends credence and rationality to interventions and therapies that are nontraditional and yet may have benefit by virtue of the interaction between the brain and the rest of the body. The connection between the mind and the body should be explored in greater detail to determine its role in healing.

Taming the Mind

The mind is similar to a child or an untamed, wandering animal. If left uncontrolled, the mind will wander and not focus or concentrate on any one particular item. You can say that the mind is naturally unfocused and disorganized.

Most of us probably think that sitting in traffic, waiting for an elevator, standing on line at the bank, or listening to music on hold over the telephone can be stressful events. But if you think about it, there's nothing intrinsically stressful about these activities. It is merely our reactions to these external events that determine whether these events are perceived as stressful (and consequently become stressful). If we can learn to control those reactions, we can also learn to control our level of stress.

For example, sitting in traffic might seem stressful to you, but it may be far less stressful to someone else. The person in the car next to you in the gridlock may be sitting quietly with her eyes closed and a serene look on her face. Why are your experiences so different when you're facing the same situation? Maybe she dislikes her job so much that she's relieved she's going to be late, or maybe she's simply found a way to say to herself, "Some things matter enough for me to get upset over, but most things don't."

That's the ultimate goal of meditation.

Fighting Back Anxiety

Because the mind has such a powerful effect on the heart and blood vessels, stress reduction usually has a beneficial effect on the body. Many anxiety-provoking situations in our environment are not anxiety provoking in and of themselves but are only perceived as such by individuals. Take the traffic jam again as an example. No one is threatening your life; no one is even confronting you in a hostile manner. There is nothing inherently dangerous or threatening about the situation, but your perception of how this mess on the freeway is going to affect the rest of your day (there's the future, rearing its ugly head) is enough to send your stress levels sky-high!

Healthy Heart Facts
Although doctors and medical scientists don't know exactly what triggers most heart attacks, some heart attacks are directly attributed to anxiety and stress. For example, after the scud missile attacks launched by Iraq against Israel the first Iraqi War, there was an increase in the number of heart attack patients in emergency rooms in parts of Israel. A similar situation occurred in California in 1994 after the Northridge earthquake: emergency rooms in California saw an increase in the number of heart-attack patients. There have also been published studies showing that the incidence of heart attacks rose in the months following 9/11, presumably due to anxiety.

Meditation How-To

Now that we've covered the many facets of stress and its causes and effects on the body, let's talk about how to use meditation to calm those feelings and to improve health.

Depending on where you live and what your life experience has been, you may hear the term meditation and dismiss it as something left over from the Free Love generation of the 1960s whose philosophies, you're proud to say, you've successfully avoided learning about.

You don't need to resign yourself to wearing tie-dyed t-shirts and growing your hair long to benefit from meditation. You only need the desire to decrease your stress level or your reaction to the occasional stressful event. These are things that most people could use a little help in achieving; the good news is that we can often help ourselves!

Meditation is simply a technique of controlling the mind. The goal of meditation is to suspend thinking and concentrate only on the present. The past and future often are responsible for our anxieties and negative emotions, so in meditation, we temporarily disregard what has already happened and what may happen down the road. Concentrating on the present gives us a sense of safety and control. In order to focus our healing thoughts and energy, we usually focus our thinking on our breathing.

> ## def•i•ni•tion
>
> **Meditation** is a method of gaining control of negative thoughts and training the mind to react in a controlled fashion. The basic principal of meditation is to focus thoughts and concentration on one item to relieve stress. This is another case of a therapy that hasn't yet been proven, and yet … it's worth a shot. At the very least, meditation puts you in a pleasant state of mind.

Reducing Anxiety

Meditation is an ancient practice that can be applied in modern times to reduce anxiety. By focusing on breathing and forcing the mind to concentrate on one task or thought, you may feel in control and perceive your environment differently. Meditation can be practiced anywhere and at any time by closing your eyes and concentrating on slow, rhythmic breathing. Over time, this technique can become perfected and utilized to achieve optimum health.

There are different ways to put yourself into a meditative state, but probably the best-known meditation style employs breathing techniques. Here's how to get yourself started:

- Sit in a comfortable position.

- Rest both hands on the knees with palms upwards. Keep your back straight and relaxed.

> ### Here's to Your Heart
>
> For thousands of years, Eastern cultures have made use of breathing exercises and techniques for focusing energy in a healing manner. Focusing energy is merely a process wherein we gain control of our emotions and their effects upon our physical health. The thinking is that controlling negative emotions may improve physical well-being.

Here's to Your Heart _____

Focusing and concentrating on your breathing will relieve stress and refresh your mental outlook. With relaxation techniques, your mental stress level can be reduced and your heart and blood vessel health can be improved.

◆ Close your eyes, and keep your head level and facing forward.

◆ Concentrate on your breathing, counting slowly from one to five, with even inhalations and even exhalations.

◆ Imagine your breath traveling as energy from all around body, through the legs, through the abdomen, the chest, and finally, out of the head. This process of energy flow should be repeated many times.

Stay focused on your breathing! When your mind wanders, redirect it toward your breathing.

It sounds as if there's nothing to this meditating business, and that anyone should be able to do it, but just try it and you'll see how difficult it is to stay focused on nothing except your inhalations and exhalations! We all have so many worries and concerns in our lives, it's tough to concentrate on (almost) nothing at all!

Aim for 5 to 30 minutes of meditation each day, and you'll see how reigning in the mind can have positive effects for every other aspect of your life!

Healthy Heart Facts

Many people who practice meditation choose to sit cross-legged on the floor, but this position might become difficult to maintain after a prolonged period. Because you don't want pains and strains to break your concentration, practice this position before you try meditating for the first time. If you find you just can't do it, sit in a comfortable chair— just make sure that your seating is not going to become a distraction.

Just Breathe!

The focus of meditation is to achieve a sense of inner calm using breathing and concentration as tools. Meditation may seek to control the body through relaxation techniques or to control the mind through use of the body, such as in tai chi, yoga, and martial arts.

The focus of the breathing exercise is to slowly, deliberately, and consciously meter the breathing so that inhalation and exhalation are performed in a controlled fashion.

Eastern cultures believe that the origin of the body energy is in the abdominal area, and so the central point of the breathing during meditation becomes the abdomen instead of the chest. Breathing exercises are performed to strengthen this area and gain control over your entire life.

When you realize that the sympathetic and parasympathetic nervous systems are intricately involved in breathing, it becomes easier to understand how controlling your breathing can help you gain some control over these nervous system relationships.

> **Healthy Heart Facts**
>
> The energy cultivated through this type of breathing may be used for healing. Various systems of breathing and body movements have been developed over thousands of years to harness this energy and benefit from it.

The Least You Need to Know

- ◆ There is a powerful mind and body connection wherein our thoughts, anxieties, and fears can affect the health of our hearts and blood vessels.

- ◆ The sympathetic nervous system initiates a fight-or-flight response in the body, which is how we feel when we're stressed.

- ◆ Chronic activation of the sympathetic nervous system can lead to organ failure.

- ◆ Meditation is about achieving a sense of calmness and quieting the sympathetic nervous system.

Chapter 17

Other Mind/Body Approaches

In This Chapter

- ◆ Learn about physical conditions that mental stress can cause

- ◆ Understand the placebo effect

- ◆ Get a handle on the sympathetic nervous system and what it means for your heart's health

- ◆ Discover the uses of biofeedback

- ◆ Find out how yoga can improve your mind and body!

In the last chapter, we discussed how the mind and body work together as a unit. As a result, mental stress has a powerful effect on the body, particularly on the heart and blood vessels—however, all the organs and systems of the body can be affected by the mind's reaction to stress. One system can knock another system out of balance, which can lead to another system falling out of sync. This only throws gasoline on the fire, so to speak. What perhaps began in the mind is reinforced by physical effects, making a person feel worse and worse, physically and mentally.

In this chapter, we'll talk about what can happen in the body when the mind is out of sorts, and how elevated cholesterol levels can lead to a disastrous outcome. However, we'll also talk about some more ways to relax (in the event you don't find meditation particularly helpful) and, in doing so, how to heal the body and the mind.

Mind Over Matter?

The mind has a powerful effect on many organ systems. There are several disorders that internists and specialists see with great frequency that are thought to have major psychological components.

For example, up to 20 percent of the general population experiences symptoms of *irritable bowel syndrome*. This is believed to be a functional gastrointestinal disorder wherein the central nervous system has a prominent effect on the nervous system of the gastrointestinal tract. It results in symptoms of diarrhea, constipation, incomplete evacuation, and abdominal discomfort. During a gastrointestinal work-up, a physical cause for the disorder is typically not found. However, often antidepressants may have some therapeutic benefit.

Fibromyalgia is another disorder with a strong psychological component. This is a condition characterized by widely scattered aches and pains, especially at specific locations called trigger points. The pain can be exacerbated by pressing on the trigger points. Again, upon examination, there doesn't seem to be a physical cause for the pain, but its symptoms often respond to exercise and antidepressants.

Connecting the Dots

All right, you say, but so what? So what if some people have fibromyalgia or irritable bowel syndrome? What does this have to do with cholesterol and your need to focus your mind?

Feeling physically unwell for a long period of time—whether the condition is real or created (or exaggerated) by the mind—can lead a person into a perpetual state of worry. Worry, meanwhile, can exacerbate physical feelings of pain or illness.

But there's an even more serious effect to this: a constant state of anxiety increases circulating levels of adrenaline-type compounds, which are helpful in a fight-or-flight type situation, but can also be destructive to the body when they remain elevated for long periods of time.

The Doctor Says

Adrenaline's effect on the body is a relative issue—that is to say, it can be good or bad. When a heart attack occurs, for instance, the adrenaline response may be the most important component for survival. But we may give antiadrenaline medication during the heart attack itself, because the excess adrenaline quickly becomes adverse. Often, we have to be careful to maintain a the correct level of this compound that can be both helpful and harmful.

These compounds have little adverse effect on the healthy hearts of young people who do not have elevated cholesterol or other risk factors for heart disease. However, for older folks, prolonged anxiety can wreak havoc on the body, particularly in people with elevated cholesterol levels and cholesterol deposited on the inside of the blood vessels. These people may experience an increased risk for serious health issues, such as constriction of the blood vessels. When the blood vessels in the heart constrict, the result can be chest pain or even sudden death!

Healthy Heart Facts

There are various sophisticated tests where doctors monitor the heart's electrical activity during periods of stress by subjecting patients to mental stress. The test results show that the patients' heart blood vessels constrict, impeding the flow of blood. This is a dangerous situation!

Because we realize that the mind and body are intricately connected, various techniques have been developed and used to control stress levels, some of which we'll talk about in the following sections. Just remember: the point of stress management is to reduce the adverse effects that negative thinking has on the cardiovascular system and other organ systems. Negative thoughts include those that result in depressive symptoms as well as anxiety.

Biofeedback

Biofeedback is a technique in which a person tries to control his or her *autonomic nervous system*. The autonomic nervous system controls involuntary functions, such as breathing and heart rate. For example, we don't have to remember to breathe in and breathe out on a constant basis, and we do not have to manually pump our hearts. These functions occur autonomously, or automatically. (Which is ideal, because who has time to squeeze their heart tens of thousands of times every day?)

def•i•ni•tion

Biofeedback is a technique where a person concentrates on breathing, heartbeat, and blood pressure in an attempt to consciously modify these functions. Biofeedback is plausible because it may allow us to consciously control our **autonomic nervous system**, which controls involuntary body functions such as breathing.

Breathing is controlled by a center within the brain; heartbeats, meanwhile, are regulated by the pacemaker center in the heart. These functions, though, are also affected by various other entities, such as anxiety. For example, when you're frightened, your body produces more adrenaline. This substance causes your heart to beat faster and can also increase your blood pressure.

Years ago, there was a great deal of enthusiasm for biofeedback. The technique makes sense. Essentially, you monitor your heartbeat and blood pressure continuously and consciously attempt to modify these functions. Biofeedback is a form of learning about your own body by attempting to consciously alter your unconscious activity. You can even attempt this using a biofeedback machine: when a conscious intervention causes a change in the heart beat, blood pressure, or other function, a light or other signal informs the subject that the biofeedback has been successful.

Currently, this therapy is not widely used, as there is little scientific data to support biofeedback for cardiovascular disease. However, biofeedback is used for a particular syndrome outside of cardiovascular disease. One cause of constipation in women is caused by pelvic floor dysfunction. The pelvic floor is a group of muscles through which the rectum passes. In pelvic floor dysfunction, the muscles exert pressure on the rectum. Consequently, it is more difficult for the contents of the rectum to pass. Biofeedback has had success in treating this condition.

Yoga

Yoga is a popular weapon in the stress-reducing arsenal. It seems as though yoga studios are popping up everywhere you turn, and many Hollywood stars swear by yoga as a means of staying in shape. Although yoga can certainly help to keep a body flexible and fit, it has been used for centuries as a means of quieting the mind and finding inner peace. We'll talk about the practice and the benefits of yoga in this section.

Stretching for Balance

Stretching is common to almost all physical activities. Athletes stretch before and after a game, and even mild activities, such as walking, should include a warm-up stretch. We tend to think of stretching as a way of preventing soreness and injury to our muscles, but ancient cultures viewed it as something quite different. To understand the role of stretching in yoga, it is important to understand the theory behind the role of both stretching and yoga.

Ancient cultures view all states of being as a balance between opposing forces. For example, the relative relaxation of a muscle or muscle group is determined by the opposing forces of contraction and relaxation. (The muscle can only be as relaxed as the opposing force allows it to be.) A tense muscle experiences excessive contraction instead of relaxation. To achieve relaxation, the muscle is stretched.

The point of stretching in yoga is to bring balance to the mind and the body. When the body is in balance, anxiety levels drop and the internal systems function as they should. This is the theory behind yoga and other techniques that seek to use muscle movements to achieve a sense of relaxation in the mind. The sense of relaxation in the mind may help to balance the *sympathetic and parasympathetic nervous systems*, which may, theoretically, improve health. We'll talk more about this balance in the following section.

def•i•ni•tion

The **parasympathetic nervous system** is part of the autonomic nervous system, which regulates the body's involuntary systems. The parasympathetic nervous system conserves energy, slowing things down in the body, while its counterpart, the **sympathetic nervous system**, initiates a "fight or flight" response.

Sympathetic to Your Body's Balance

We know that when the heart is healthy, there is a balance between the parasympathetic nervous system and sympathetic nervous system, wherein the parasympathetic nervous system is dominant. When the heart is diseased, however, the sympathetic nervous system steps up and takes charge. It's well-known that with increases in various markers for sympathetic nervous system overactivity, mortality due to heart disease goes up.

There are several tests that can measure the balance of sympathetic and parasympathetic nervous systems. One such test is called a *heart rate variability study*. When the heart rate

def•i•ni•tion

A **heart rate variability study** can evaluate the measure of balance between the parasympathetic and sympathetic nervous systems. If the sympathetic nervous system is dominant, this is a sign of trouble!

changes in an orderly fashion with activity, it implies that the parasympathetic and sympathetic nervous systems are balanced, as this state of increased heart rate variability is healthy. There will also be changes in the heart electrical activity called *T wave alternans*. When the T wave alternans is abnormal, there is an increase in the sympathetic nervous system activity. This imbalance is a sign of disease and is actually a warning sign for increased risk of sudden death!

The lesson to be learned is that the heart and circulatory system are continuously upgrading information and changing on a second-to-second basis relative to other functions within the body. A healthy balance between sympathetic and parasympathetic activity implies a healthy heart. The balance between the two systems also implies a healthy nervous and cardiovascular system. Practicing yoga can actually help to achieve this balance between the body's systems.

It's remarkable that our culture has only recently taken this state of harmony into consideration, because this has been a central facet in many cultures and systems of medicine for thousands of years!

Balanced Breath

Breathing also assumes a role in yoga. Similar to the opposition of contraction and relaxation that characterizes muscle states, breathing is characterized by opposite forces: inhalation and exhalation.

Ancient cultures believed that restoring control of breathing may restore one's health and may be an avenue for achieving optimum health. Yoga combines deliberate postures and breathing techniques to achieve stress reduction. These breathing techniques use body movements to improve mental activity, and are slow, deliberate, and metered. Inhalations and exhalations are equal in length and are counted. Typically, you'll inhale and exhale to the count of 5 or 10 while concentrating on the execution of the various movements.

The Doctor Says

Conditions such as advanced heart failure, obesity, lung disease, and neurological diseases may be characterized by abnormal breathing.

Other Relaxation Exercises

Controlled breathing is a powerful method of stress reduction and is often included in a stress-reduction regimen. For example, martial-arts experts are trained to focus on their breathing and combine controlled breathing and controlled movement to focus their energy.

Ancient cultures believe the combination of breathing and movements can harness energy to be utilized in a healing fashion as well as for martial-arts purposes. Martial-arts experts further employ meditation and focusing techniques to further apply their skills.

Tai Chi

An effective way to utilize controlled breathing is in combination with other techniques, such as imagery, meditation, or various martial arts techniques. An example of a martial art that may be used for relaxation is *tai chi chuan*, which is a form of soft martial arts; it combines thought, medicine, and martial arts techniques to achieve relaxation.

Tai chi is a slow martial arts style that seeks to achieve balance and harmony. Energy is gathered up and circulated through the body in combination with slow and deliberate inhalations and exhalations. The flow of energy and the performance of the motion is believed to improve health.

Kung Fu

Another example of relaxation exercise is a soft type of kung fu. In this style of kung fu, the martial arts practitioner performs various movements combined with controlled inhalations and exhalations to gather energy. This energy or force is called *gingh*.

Soft kung fu experts practice gathering this energy and harnessing it for healing purposes. The relative health benefits of these systems have not been adequately studied in a rigorous, scientific fashion. But it certainly is interesting to think about how medical technologies can measure the relative balance between the sympathetic and parasympathetic nervous systems and the role of this balance in health, and then compare that with how these ancient systems have sought to achieve a similar sense of balance for centuries.

Healthy Heart Facts

Various relaxation techniques that are rooted in ancient cultures are still being used today. For example, imagery is a technique that athletes utilize to envision their goal and to achieve relaxation. Similarly, modern athletes meditate and control their breathing prior to an athletic competition to achieve relaxation and control over their bodies.

The Least You Need to Know

- The mind and body are intricately connected. The health of one affects the health of the other.

- The placebo effect is a powerful indicator of the mind's control over our health.

- Biofeedback was popular years ago, but has shown no evidence of health benefits from its use.

- Relaxation techniques, such as yoga, can have a calming effect on the body's fight-or-flight system.

Part 4

Medications and Other Natural Remedies

After discussing cholesterol-lowering medications with their doctors, many people walk out of the office feeling confused, to say the least. They've just been bombarded with a lot of information, and the names of the medications alone are sometimes enough to shut a patient down mentally. Then there are dosages, side effects, intended effects, and drug interactions to consider … no wonder people are feeling overwhelmed!

Pharmacists—professionals in the field of medicine—learn this stuff over a matter of *years!* Part 4 of this book talks about common medications used for the purpose of lowering cholesterol levels, as well as some natural supplements that some people swear by. We also look at some new therapies that are being studied and put into practice right now.

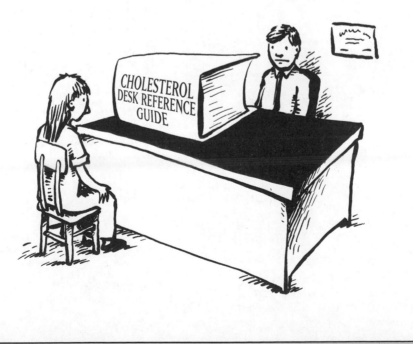

Chapter 18

Understanding Statins

In This Chapter

- ◆ Learn about statins
- ◆ Understand how statins work with the liver to lower cholesterol
- ◆ Read about the pleiotropic effects of statins
- ◆ Arm yourself with knowledge about possible side effects of statins

When faced with elevated cholesterol levels that do not respond to modified diet and increased activity levels, your doctor may recommend using a medication to help bring those cholesterol numbers down. One of the most popular class of drugs in use today is called statins. In this chapter, we'll talk about the rather amazing effects that can be achieved by using statins (in conjunction with diet and exercise, of course) as a means of lowering cholesterol. They also happen to be safe drugs, which makes them an ideal choice for almost anyone.

What Are Statins?

Over the years, various categories of medication have been created to decrease cholesterol. Using medication for cholesterol disorders seeks to

def•i•ni•tion

One class of medications that doctors use to treat cholesterol disorders is called **statins**. These are safe drugs whose primary mechanism of action is to remove LDL from the bloodstream.

achieve several goals. One goal of any cholesterol-lowering medication is to decrease LDL, decrease triglycerides, and increase HDL. The most successful group of medications for this purpose is called *statins*. Statins not only reduce cholesterol but also decrease mortality due to heart disease. Although some of the benefits of statins are still being debated, these drugs have been one of the most successful categories of medication ever developed!

The reason why the statins have been so successful is that their use in individuals with high cholesterol (with and without heart diseases) has been associated with a reduced mortality because of heart disease. In other words, when people who have heart disease are given statins, they will most likely live longer. One primary benefit of the statins is reduction of heart attack mortality by reducing fatal and nonfatal myocardial infarction (the medical term for heart attack). The statins also prevent rupture of plaque.

Healthy Heart Facts

As a group, heart patients who take statins live longer. What this means is that perhaps not every single person who takes the medication will have a prolonged life, but most will. To find out if you're a candidate for a statin drug, talk to your doctor. He or she will take a look at your LDL level and your risk factors and decide whether you might benefit from this class of medications.

The pharmaceutical industry's major focus on statin development is a high degree of LDL reduction. Other benefits of statins include HDL elevation and triglyceride lowering.

Statins have been so successful because they interfere with the natural history of heart disease in people who have elevated cholesterol and other risk factors for heart disease. Individuals with heart-disease risk factors are likely to die of heart disease at some point in their lives. Statins enter the body and reduce the likelihood of heart attack and stroke, and thus also reduce the chance of death from these conditions.

A Statin by Any Other Name ...

There are many different types of statins. They differ from one another in potency; however, the key to using statins is to use the greatest dose. So whichever statin a doctor decides to use, the trend in medical practice over the years has been to increase the dose; this trend toward the use of higher doses has paralleled the trend toward driving LDL levels as low as possible.

Although higher doses are associated with an increased risk of side effects, the *risk/ benefit ratio* is in favor of using higher doses in most patients, unless there is a significant risk of side effects. The greater the baseline patient risk, the greater the benefit with higher doses of statins. So the greater the risk for heart disease and the higher the cholesterol, the greater the motive to use higher doses of statins.

def•i•ni•tion

You may hear your doctor talk about **risk/benefit ratio** when discussing medications or other treatment options. This means that your doctor weighs the benefits of a particular course of treatment against the possibility of a negative outcome. If you're far more likely to benefit from a medication than to suffer an adverse effect, the benefits outweigh the risks.

Commonly Used Statins

The most popular and frequently used statins include these drugs:

- Lipitor (generic name: atorvastatin)

- Zocor (simvastatin)

- Pravachol (pravastatin)

- Crestor (rosuvastatin)

 The Doctor Says

Statins are remarkable drugs; however, the best results for reducing LDL levels are achieved using a combination of medication, exercise and a healthy diet.

Other statins include Mevacor (lovastatin) and Lescol (fluvastatin).

It really doesn't matter which statin you use, as long as you take the medication on a consistent basis and have your liver and muscle enzymes evaluated regularly. (We discuss the reasons for this shortly.) You should also be proactive in following your LDL response; you might just be surprised at the results. A recent study that sought to determine how low to reduce LDL found that there was no adverse effect when LDL was reduced to just 30 mg/dl! This is remarkable, as typically statins reduce LDL by only a percentage. (We have to keep in mind that to drive LDL to less than 30, high doses are likely required.)

How Statins Work

Your liver has LDL receptors are embedded within the membranes of the liver cells. These molecules attach to LDL circulating within the blood and remove the LDL particles. A good way to imagine the LDL receptors is as little swimming-pool filters. Envision the swimming pool as your bloodstream. LDL receptors are filters that remove large particles from the bloodstream, in the same way a pool filter gets rid of bugs and leaves. In the case of the human body, the LDL receptors remove LDL from the blood. Statins increase the activity of these receptors, which remove more LDL from the blood.

The number of LDL receptors sitting atop the liver cells is determined genetically and modified by environmental influences. (In simpler terms, you have a given number of receptors at birth and that number can change due to things such as your diet and cholesterol levels.) So different people are born with different numbers of LDL receptors in their liver cells. In circumstances of excess cholesterol consumption, the liver cells can make more receptors and perch them on top of the cell membranes in greater numbers, so that the LDL can be removed from the circulation at a greater rate! (Pretty amazing, isn't it?)

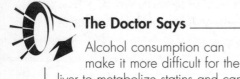

The Doctor Says

Alcohol consumption can make it more difficult for the liver to metabolize statins and can lead to toxic levels in the body.

When someone takes a statin, the drug stimulates the liver cells to make more LDL receptors and, as a result, remove more LDL from the bloodstream. And of course, when more LDL is removed from the blood by the liver, less is left over to deposit within the arteries in the form of plaque. Although there is much debate about the various benefits of takings statins, it's clear that statins reduce LDL and reduce mortality from heart disease.

Pleasing Pleiotropic Effects

Some doctors and medical scientists believe that statins have multiple beneficial effects, or what we call *pleiotropic effects*. For example, in addition to removing LDL from the bloodstream, there is data that statins may also improve the overall health of the blood vessels.

A particularly interesting effect of statins is called *myocardial regeneration*. When someone has a heart attack, he or she loses heart muscle; in fact, the term for this is *heart muscle death* (which doesn't exactly paint a hopeful picture of this person's future).

For decades it was believed that when someone had a heart attack and lost heart muscle, the muscle would not regenerate or rebuild itself; it would be replaced by scar tissue.

Let's back up for just a second to consider what we're talking about. Think about an injury where the tip of someone's finger is severed by a knife. The fingertip will never regenerate the missing part. Now, imagine a therapy where a group of cells could travel to the finger and divide into various cell types that could reestablish the fingertip—now, keep in mind that these rescue cells would have to divide into many different types of cells that could re-create bone cells, muscle cells, nerves, and so on. That would really be something, wouldn't it, if one type of cell could fix other cells?

Well, it turns out that such a cell exists. It's found in low numbers in the blood and is sometimes found dormant in heart muscle. It's called a *progenitor cell*, and when it's stimulated, it has the ability to regrow dead heart muscle. Remarkably, statins stimulate this cell type! And although taking a statin will not completely regrow new heart muscle cells, it provides a powerful stimulus to these cells and may unlock a mechanism to encourage heart muscle regrowth to a greater extent.

def•i•ni•tion

When a therapy has multiple benefits, doctors sometimes say that it has **pleiotropic** effects. For instance, statins work to lower LDL, improve the overall condition of the blood vessels, and help stimulate **progenitor cells,** a type of cell that helps to rebuild damaged cells. Progenitor cells help to stimulate **myocardial regeneration,** or the rebuilding of heart muscle lost during a heart attack.

Turning Down the (Plaque) Volume

Recent investigations into statins have demonstrated that the greater the dose, the greater the reduction in plaque volume.

Ultrasound studies of the effects of statins have shown that the amount of plaque on the inside of blood vessels is reduced with statin use. In addition to reducing overall plaque volume, there is a reduction in the likelihood of the plaque rupturing. And you know by now that a reduced likelihood of plaque rupture translates into a reduced risk of an occlusive blood clot and consequent heart attack.

Is There Anything Statins Don't Do?

In addition to the amazing effects just mentioned, there is evidence that statins do even more. For example …

- Heart failure may be attenuated by the use of statins, (which, in turn, prolongs the life of the heart failure patient).

- Statins may also decrease macular degeneration, a deterioration of the eye.

- Statins reduce the likelihood of stroke as well, by decreasing the rupture and subsequent blood clot formation that takes place over plaques that are located in the arteries that deliver blood to the brain (called the carotid arteries).

- There is evidence that statins may be beneficial for heart-attack patients immediately following a heart attack, perhaps even for people who have normal cholesterol levels.

So…what's the catch? There really isn't one. Statins are one of the safest drug categories and cause few side effects. We talk about these unlikely side effects in the following section.

Major Side Effects to Know About

A small percentage of patients (less than 1 percent) have shown liver-enzyme elevations and muscle problems in conjunction with statin use. Now, because the liver is such an important organ, we're going to talk about its functions, so that you can better understand the risks involved with taking a statin or any medicine that may cause liver-enzyme elevations.

Statins and Elevated Enzymes

The liver performs many functions in the body. It synthesizes various substances that are necessary for life; it also detoxifies various substances before they're sent off to be excreted by the kidneys and urine.

When the liver is exposed to a drug that causes it harm, it may release enzymes as an indication of injury. For example, excessive alcohol consumption can lead to an elevation of liver enzymes because the liver has enzymes that break down alcohol into simpler components. As the liver's alcohol-detoxifying activity is stressed because of excess alcohol consumption, it may release enzymes into the blood that can be readily measured. When the liver is injured by liver virus (hepatitis), it may also release *enzymes*.

Some people may experience an elevation of their liver enzymes when taking a statin. Most of the time, if the elevation is minor, the physician may choose to continue the statin because the risk/benefit ratio is in favor of preventing heart disease because of the statin.

def•i•ni•tion

An **enzyme** is a protein that is used to help promote a particular reaction in a cell as part of the cell's metabolism. Elevated enzyme levels may indicate injury or damage in a particular organ.

Many people are frightened of the rare possibility of liver damage due to statins and thus don't take the medication. These individuals incur a much higher risk of heart disease from not taking the statin than having liver problems if they took the drug. The decision as to whether to continue the statin should be left up to the physician. These side effects can be minimized by follow-up blood work that monitors your liver enzymes. When statins are administered under a physician's care, they are remarkably safe (maybe even as safe as aspirin).

In addition, because statins can increase muscle enzymes, a physician should evaluate these enzymes on a regular basis. Any out-of-the-ordinary aches and pains should trigger a visit to the physician to be certain there is no toxicity due to the statin. A person will typically experience muscle soreness when the muscle enzymes increase. This soreness is usually out of proportion to any physical activity recently performed.

The Doctor Says

Some people may have an elevated risk for liver enzyme elevations. These individuals may have liver disease in addition to heart disease. One should, therefore, use these medications carefully when liver disease exists. The decision to use a statin in a patient with liver disease should be made by a physician.

Any muscle soreness or tenderness, even if minor, should be reported to a physician. Serious muscle enzyme elevation can lead to significant amounts of protein in the urine and the possibility of kidney failure.

Combination Therapies

Often, a patient will have severe cholesterol abnormalities. A patient who has had a heart attack and who has abnormal cholesterol levels while taking a statin will need to have another medication added. This type of *combination therapy* can further improve cholesterol levels, but it increases the risk for side effects.

When cholesterol remains abnormal on treatment, two common classes of medications that are added to statins include *fibric acids* and *niacin*. Both can increase the risk for liver-enzyme and muscle-enzyme elevations. The reason combination therapy increases this risk is that one enzyme may be responsible for breaking down both substances.

> **Healthy Heart Facts**
>
> Baycol (cerivastatin) is a statin that was removed from the market several years ago due to multiple episodes of muscle breakdown and consequent renal (kidney) toxicity. In almost all cases, the toxicity was seen in patients who took cerivastatin and another medication, such as a fibric acid.

When the second drug is added, the enzyme that breaks down the statin is saturated. Think of the enzyme as being overworked; it just can't do any more than it's already doing. Consequently, statin levels in the bloodstream rise into a toxic range.

Although the risk of satin use is small when used alone, the risk does go up when statins are combined with other medications that lower cholesterol. If your doctor recommends using multiple medications, he should also assess your liver and muscle enzymes on a regular basis.

Minor Side Effects to Know About

Besides the side effects relating to liver and muscle enzyme elevations, there are few other side effects related to taking statins. Sometimes, people may experience some mild gastrointestinal discomfort, a rash, or a headache. Overall, though, the statins are extremely well tolerated with few side effects. So in addition to their wonderful and plentiful positive effects, their lack of negative effects makes statins the drug of choice for many doctors and their patients. They can be used in patients with few risk factors as well as in patients with many risk factors—both groups have shown benefit from using these drugs!

> **Healthy Heart Facts**
>
> How does a doctor determine which patients should be taking statins? It's a process of evaluation—namely, evaluation of risk factors. Your doctor will take a look at whether you have diagnosed heart disease, elevated LDL levels, and other risk factors. From there, he'll determine whether statin use is appropriate and likely to be beneficial.

This drug category is a highly successful group of medications because they reduce mortality due to heart attacks in a dose-dependent manner and they have a good safety profile. The statins are truly miracle drugs.

The Least You Need to Know

- ◆ Statins are a highly effective and safe group of medications.

- ◆ LDL reduction is the primary way the LDLs work to improve health.

- ◆ The greater the statin dose, the greater the LDL reduction.

- ◆ There is an increased risk for liver and muscle toxicity with higher doses of statins.

- ◆ A physician should regularly evaluate the muscle and liver enzymes of patients taking statins.

Other Cholesterol-Lowering Medications

In This Chapter

◆ Understand the many medications available for reducing cholesterol levels

◆ Know why early and aggressive intervention for elevated LDL is becoming the norm

◆ Learn why some drugs are more effective than others

◆ See the potential side effects of these drugs

Currently, the statins are the first drugs of choice in most instances of cholesterol elevation that don't respond to a change in diet and activity level. However, a small percentage of people (less than 1%) cannot tolerate statins. Some will experience major side effects, such as marked elevation of liver enzymes or muscle enzymes; others may suffer from more minor side effects that are not likely life-threatening but may be a nuisance.

Fortunately, there are other drug therapies that can be used for those who don't tolerate statins well. Bile acid sequestrants or resins, niacin, fibric acids, and ezetimide are all viable drug therapies that may be used in place of statins with somewhat different effects on the lipid subfractions. We talk about each of these alternatives in this chapter.

Niacin

Niacin is actually a B vitamin. When used in low doses, it acts as a vitamin; when used in higher doses, it acts as a pharmaceutical and reduces LDL, reduces triglycerides, and elevates HDL.

Why don't we use niacin for every person with elevated cholesterol? It must be readily available, and because it falls into the vitamin category, niacin is probably somewhat inexpensive, right? As we'll discuss in this section, niacin isn't right for everyone.

Oh, My Burning Cheeks!

Niacin tends to be poorly tolerated. It causes an uncomfortable sensation of flushing (burning of the cheeks) that becomes more prominent when dosages are escalated rapidly. Therefore, niacin therapy has to be started slowly, and doses should be increased gradually. Flushing can be prevented by taking an aspirin tablet, 325 mg, or Tylenol thirty minutes prior to taking your niacin.

> **The Doctor Says**
>
> Niacin's tendency to elevate blood sugar may be a concern when a person has metabolic syndrome, because this condition is characterized by insulin resistance and a prediabetic state. For more details on metabolic syndrome, read Chapter 4.

Niacin also has other multiple side effects to think about, such as liver toxicity and elevated blood sugar. Niacin is also thought to initiate diabetes or worsen elevated blood sugar in people who already have diabetes.

Caution: Niacin in Use!

Muscle and liver toxicity may become major concerns when niacin is added to other medications used to treat elevated cholesterol; as a result, niacin must be used cautiously when combined with other medications, especially other cholesterol-reducing medications such as statins and fibric acids.

Niacin is available in various time-release formulas, which, in theory, is terrific: niacin continues working in the body long after you've taken the pill. The benefit of sustained-release niacin is that fewer dosages are required and the flushing may be alleviated somewhat. However, using the time-release formulas may increase risk of liver toxicity, which is obviously a significant concern.

Don't Mess with the Doses!

Only a physician can titrate, or adjust, dosages of medications and base their use upon a risk-stratification process.

What does this mean to you? Well, the higher your risk of heart disease, the more compelling the reason for your physician to start you on a cholesterol-reducing medication, which will most likely be a statin. But remember, although statins are amazing drugs, not everyone has great luck then. Sometimes cholesterol doesn't drop as much as we'd like it to, even with statin use. When cholesterol continues to be elevated after statins have been started, doctors usually feel the need to add a second cholesterol-reducing therapy, such as niacin.

Here's to Your Heart

Niacin is usually started as 100 mg twice per day and gradually increased over several weeks to 1.5 to 3 grams per day. Again, any flushing that occurs can be alleviated by taking an aspirin tablet, 325 mg, or Tylenol 30 minutes before taking niacin.

Healthy Heart Facts

Niacin has a powerful reductive effect on triglycerides and LDL. Niacin also raises HDL. However, niacin has never been shown to reduce cardiovascular mortality in the same way as the statins. Consequently, statins remain the first choice for prevention of cardiovascular events.

Bile Acid Resins

The statins became available by prescription in the early to mid-1990s and revolutionized cholesterol reduction therapy. Prior to the advent of the statins, the only cholesterol-reducing medications available were niacin, fibric acids (which we'll talk about later in this chapter), and resins, which we discuss in this section.

You might have heard this class of medications referred to as bile acid sequestrants. For the sake of ease, most doctors refer to these medications simply as resins (and that's what I will call them during this discussion!).

Right This Way, Cholesterol ...

Resins interfere with the cycling of cholesterol from the liver to the digestive tract and back. Resins set up a sort of phony detour for cholesterol, except instead of rerouting cholesterol to somewhere else in the body, resins show cholesterol the door. As a result of the resins' interface with cholesterol, cholesterol is excreted from the digestive tract in the stool. By blocking the reabsorption of cholesterol, resin lowers cholesterol levels.

Studies of resins showed a decrease in cholesterol and a decrease in heart attacks but not a decrease in mortality. When the statins became available, they demonstrated a reduction in mortality, making them the first choice of medication for lowering cholesterol levels.

Stuck on the Pharmacy Shelf

The original resins are rarely used today. They were taken several times a day in the form of packets that were mixed with juice or water, they caused flatulence and abdominal discomfort, and they were not as tolerable as the statins.

> **The Doctor Says**
>
> One group of individuals for whom resins may not be useful are people with elevated triglycerides, as these medications can elevate triglycerides further.

However, one new and well-tolerated resin called colesevelam has emerged. It's nearly devoid of side effects, because the resins are not absorbed, as they were with colesevelam's predecessors. The resins now remain in the gastrointestinal tract, where they perform their duties without causing any gastrointestinal upset.

Fibric Acid Derivatives

Fibric acids are used to lower triglycerides and elevate HDL. When compared with the data we have on statins, the information in favor of fibric acid use for reduction of cardiovascular events such as heart attack and stroke are much less encouraging.

Prior to the introduction of the statins, fibric acids were used by themselves. Although they reduced LDL and triglycerides and raised HDL and also showed a reduction in heart attacks and strokes, they were not associated with a reduction in total mortality until many years after patients had started on these drugs. The early studies actually suspected an increase in noncardiovascular mortality despite positive effects on the cholesterol level and its subfractions, making it a less attractive drug of choice when the super-effective statins came into play.

Fibric Acid Facts

The major fibric acid is gemfibrozil, which has been shown to reduce the likelihood of cardiovascular trouble, even though it provides only a modest elevation in HDL. Basically, the people who are most likely to benefit from this drug are already at high risk for heart disease and have a low HDL level. When cholesterol subfractions remain abnormal after statins have been started and adjusted to higher doses, a doctor may give some consideration to starting a fibric acid such as gemfibrozil.

This isn't simply a matter of adding another medication to help cholesterol levels, however. Fibric acids are associated with toxicities primarily when they're combined with statins and niacin. A doctor must monitor the liver and muscle enzyme levels on a regular basis as the risk for toxicity rises, especially with higher dosages.

One example of a particular dangerous combination of a statin and a fibric acid is cerivastatin and gemfibrozil. Using these medications together results in severe muscle enzyme elevations in a relatively high percentage of patients. In case studies, the muscle enzymes were so elevated in some patients that renal (kidney) toxicity occurred. Interestingly, the combination of cerivastatin and fenofibrate was not associated with as high an incidence of muscle toxicity. Cerivastatin has since been removed from the market and is no longer available.

Here's to Your Heart

One fibric acid that has recently been introduced in the United States is called fenofibrate. Compared with other fibric acids, it is associated with a lower incidence of adverse effects when combined with a statin. But again, because of the possibility of toxicity, a physician must closely follow liver and muscle enzymes whenever these medications are used.

Dangerous Interactions

The interaction of statins and fibric acids is quite complex. Some statins are associated with a greater incidence of liver and muscle enzyme elevations when combined with a fibric acid primarily because of a difference in the metabolism of the statin drug by the liver. When these drugs are taken in combination, the fibric acid may interfere with the statin breakdown by the liver, elevating its concentration in the blood to dangerous levels that are associated with a greater risk for muscle toxicity.

Whatever the combination, and whatever the case of toxicity, it is important that a doctor monitor these enzyme levels in a patient who is taking both classes of these drugs!

Cholesterol Absorption Inhibitors

By blocking the absorption of cholesterol into the body, it seems as though the problem would be solved. But it's not that easy (if it were, I wouldn't be writing this book). In this section, I'll talk about a dramatic way to prevent cholesterol absorption, and I'll also get into one of the newest medications available, one that's showing great promise.

Surgical Removal of Your Cholesterol Problem

When I talked about the resins earlier in this chapter, I said that they take up residence in the gastrointestinal tract, preventing the absorption of cholesterol into the body. Well, there's a surgical procedure that can provide the same basic service. During this surgery, a portion of the intestine that absorbs cholesterol is removed. The operation is successful at reducing cholesterol and preventing heart attacks.

Though it may seem like the ultimate quick fix, the surgery is not common. It was done before the introduction of statins. It works, but it's really not a useful treatment for elevated cholesterol. I bring it up here for its historical role and because it's also an example the mechanism of action of the bile acid sequestrants. The bile acid sequestrants prevent the reabsorption of cholesterol in the intestine by binding to it, so we no longer have to think about cutting anything out of you to improve your cholesterol levels!

The Newest Absorption Drug on the Block

Ezetimide belongs to a new class of medications that prevent absorption of cholesterol, much like the resins do. However, ezetimide works in a different way. The resins prevent the reabsorption of cholesterol. Some cholesterol from the liver makes it to the bile, which is secreted into the intestine. Some of this cholesterol is excreted in the stool. Some is reabsorbed and transported back to the liver for reuse. In comparison, the mechanism of action of ezetimide is not completely known. We know that it prevents the absorption of cholesterol from food at the level of the intestinal cells, as opposed to blocking its reabsorption.

Ezetimide has a low incidence of side effects, which makes it safe; it's well tolerated by most people. Ezetimide can be used alone, but is often combined with a statin to enhance LDL reduction in patients whose LDL continues to be elevated even when they're on high-dose statins, or for patients who experience side effects from statins.

> **Healthy Heart Facts**
>
> In addition to lowering LDL, eze-timide reduces triglyceride levels and elevates HDL. Although it's clear that statins reduce mortality due to heart disease, ezetimide's effects on heart attacks, strokes, and mortality are not yet known.

LDL Filtering or Apheresis

Situations where LDL remains high (several hundred mg/dl) are uncommon, but when they happen, they are, of course, very dangerous. When LDL levels are extremely high, as they may be in certain inherited disorders, the LDL reduction achieved by maximum doses of medications such as statins and bile acid sequestrants may not be enough.

An experimental technique has been devised where LDL is removed from the blood by a filtration process. This technique is modeled after other procedures where cells or substances in the blood may be removed from the body, cleaned up, and sent back in. This technology has now become available in certain institutions that have the appropriate equipment, and is called *LDL filtration*, or *apheresis*.

> **def•i•ni•tion**
>
> **LDL filtration**, or **apheresis**, is a technique by which LDL is physically removed from the bloodstream using a machine that separates the LDL and some other adverse cholesterol subfractions using columns of beads that bind the LDL and other components, such as VLDL, or very low density lipoproteins.

Think of LDL filtration like dialysis. The blood is removed from the body and run through a machine that essentially filters out the LDL. The blood is returned to the body with a dramatic reduction on LDL. The procedure is performed every two to three weeks and takes about two to four hours.

Who Needs It?

The primary use for physical removal of LDL from the bloodstream or LDL apheresis is for people who have genetic defects of LDL receptors. These people are unable to remove LDL from the bloodstream naturally, even if they follow every recommendation from their doctor for reducing cholesterol levels. These people have extremely elevated LDL levels. We're not talking about slight elevations; we're talking about levels that may reach 500 mg/dl and higher! People with these types of LDL elevations develop early atherosclerosis and sometimes have heart attacks at a young age. (Individuals with LDL-receptor deficiencies may even develop heart attacks in their teens!)

Although the use of apheresis is primarily in helping people with genetic defects at this time, there has been interest in using this process in people with less critical LDL elevations. The role of LDL apheresis may very well expand to include people with more modest LDL levels in the future.

Aspirin

Although aspirin does not have any cholesterol-reducing effects, it is a key medication for reducing the risk for heart attack and stroke. Yes, that inexpensive little white pill you've taken for years and years for your headaches can actually help improve the health of your cardiovascular system!

There is no doubt that aspirin reduces heart attack and stroke risk in individuals who already have known heart disease or risk factors for heart disease. There is some debate, however, concerning the exact dose of aspirin that is useful. This has been a hotly debated issue for the last couple of decades. The recommended dose is between 81 and 325 mg per day, depending on the situation. For example:

- For a person having a heart attack, the recommended dosage is 325 mg, chewed.

- Someone who is in the emergency room receiving clot-busting therapy would be given 162 mg/day.

- A patient who has had a heart attack is often given 162 mg/day while in the hospital.

- People with a history of heart disease should take 81 mg/day.

Healthy Heart Facts

Most people who have elevated cholesterol or otherwise abnormal cholesterol panels will benefit from aspirin. The decision as to whether to use aspirin, however, should be made by your physician, because its risk-to-benefit ratio needs to be evaluated in regards to your health.

The actual dosage isn't as important as you'd think. Experts quibble all the time over how much aspirin is enough and how much is too much. The most important thing is for people with heart disease to *listen to what their doctors tell them and to take the aspirin*, regardless of the dosage. We'll talk about aspirin's blood thinning mechanism later in this section.

Aspirin's Astounding Effects

The data concerning aspirin and heart health is robust and definitive. (Over 100,000 patients have been studied in clinical trials over the years!) The benefits of aspirin include reduction in stroke and heart attack in people who are at risk for these events and in those who have already suffered a previous heart attack or stroke. Interestingly, the benefits of aspirin are proportional to the baseline risk. In other words, people who are at higher risk for heart attack, stroke, and death due to heart disease will benefit the most from aspirin therapy.

Aspirin plays a major role in reducing the damage that may occur when someone has a heart attack. When a heart attack occurs, the plaque on the inside of a heart artery ruptures, leading to a blood clot in the blood vessel. This blood clot can obstruct the flow of blood and cause loss of heart muscle. This leads to chest pain, heart failure, and electrical-impulse problems that can result in sudden death. When a heart attack occurs, then, the most important task is to open the blood vessel up and allow blood to circulate down that blocked artery.

> **Healthy Heart Facts**
>
> One powerful effect of aspirin is its ability to open up heart arteries that are filled with blood clots in the throes of a heart attack. One study conducted in the late 1980s revealed that aspirin, taken within the first 24 hours of a heart attack, was almost as effective as other clot-busting medications.

Clot-Buster!

Let's talk about that blood clot for a minute. A blood clot is made up of strands of fibers called *fibrin strands*. These strands may be compared to a woven fabric; they're cross-linked and enmeshed with each other. Trapped within the fibers are platelets, which encourage blood clotting by sticking to each other and to the blood vessel wall. The platelets can be prevented from sticking to each other by administering anti-platelet medications. One medication that falls into this category is aspirin!

def•i•ni•tion

A blood clot is composed of **fibrin strands,** which are fibers that enmesh themselves and trap platelets inside of them. Aspirin is one medication that helps to prevent clots from forming and/or stops clots from growing larger. This gives the body time to set its own anti-platelet mechanism into action; it also allows time for clot-busting drugs (like those given in the emergency room) to take effect.

Side Effects of Aspirin

Aspirin is remarkably safe. The most serious side effect of aspirin is the risk of bleeding complications; this risk increases with higher doses. People with preexisting bleeding disorders may experience a greater risk of bleeding with aspirin use. (Someone with an ulcer, for example, may be at a higher risk for bleeding when taking aspirin.) People who have serious medical problems and other chronic medical conditions may experience greater risks as well. For example, the elderly are more likely to incur bleeding risk due to aspirin (and yet, the elderly are most likely to benefit from aspirin).

Don't try to medicate yourself with aspirin. The issues regarding aspirin use may be rather complex and should be discussed with a physician. Rarely, some people may have a hypersensitivity to aspirin that would contraindicate its use. Sometimes, platelets may be dysfunctional and unable to participate in the clotting that is needed on a day-to-day basis. As a result, people with clotting disorders that increase bleeding risk may not benefit from aspirin. Sometimes, use of aspirin is associated with bleeding risk when it's taken with other medications. Play it safe and talk to your doctor about whether a daily aspirin will be beneficial to your health.

The Doctor Says

The major problem associated with aspirin-related bleeding is spontaneous bleeding in the brain and gastrointestinal tract. Thankfully, these are rare events, occurring mostly in people who have had previous incidents of bleeding in these areas. Surgeons prefer to operate on patients who have been aspirin-free for 7 to 10 days, since aspirin can make it difficult to control bleeding after surgery.

Benefits of Cholesterol-Reducing Medications

The main goal of cholesterol reduction in this day and age is to reduce LDL to the lowest levels possible; this translates into decreasing LDL to 70 mg/dl or lower in people who have heart disease. This goal may drop even further as we glean new information from current studies.

It has become clear that heart disease must be prevented early; to that end, LDL cholesterol reduction should begin early and include an aggressive plan of attack, including medications when the situation warrants them. One thing we're learning is that people who have risk factors for heart disease (such as diabetes, high blood pressure, obesity, and high cholesterol) usually already have heart disease, which puts them at a higher risk for stroke, heart attack, and sudden death. Reducing cholesterol is obviously one way to prevent a myriad of health problems, and using medications to achieve a significant reduction is sometimes the best (and only) option.

A important topic for the population in general (and for individuals, in particular) concerns the achievement of LDL goals. Various health agencies have advocated reducing LDL using diet, exercise, and medication, but in reality, these goals are seldom met in clinical practice. One reason for this failure to achieve LDL targets is that people frequently start a cholesterol-reduction program and lose interest over time.

Long-term benefits can only be achieved by sticking with a cholesterol-reducing program—this isn't something you can adhere to intermittently. In the long run, the advantages to your health are well worth all of your efforts!

> **Healthy Heart Facts**
>
> As people who are at risk for heart disease merge with people who have known (or established) heart disease, goals for LDL reduction may decrease even further for both groups.

Side Effects

Let's just to cut to the chase here and list the most common cholesterol-reducing medications and their side effects for easy reference:

Statins/Major side effects:

Elevated muscle and liver enzymes, muscle and liver toxicity with higher enzymes elevations. Lower enzyme elevations can sometimes be watched by the doctor. It depends on how urgent it is that an individual has his cholesterol controlled. For example, an individual with a recent heart attack and a very high LDL should have his LDL reduced, in general, even if there are mild elevations in the liver enzymes. However, this should only be performed under a physician's supervision and clinical judgment.

Statins/Minor side effects:

Nausea, diarrhea, rash, constipation, headache

Fibric acids/Major side effects:

Muscle and liver enzymes elevations, especially with combination therapy

Fibric acids/Minor side effects:

Increased lithogenicity of bile (greater likelihood of forming stones; not highly common or clinically significant)

Rash, nausea, diarrhea

Niacin/Major side effects:

Muscle and liver enzyme elevation, especially when used in combination with statins or fibric acids

Niacin/Minor side effects:

Elevated blood sugar, flushing, increased uric acid and increased risk for gout in those who have had previous attacks, migraine, peptic ulcer, skin hyperpigmentation (increased skin pigmentation), rapid heartbeat

Bile Acid Sequestrants/Major side effects:

None

Bile Acid Sequestrants/Minor side effects:

Diarrhea, gastrointestinal upset, nausea

Ezetimide/Major side effects:

None

Ezetimide/Minor side effects:

Gastrointestinal upset, nausea, diarrhea

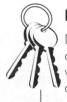

Here's to Your Heart _____

Newer cholesterol-reducing drugs include colesevelam and ezetimide. Colesevelam is a new member of an older class of medications that is not absorbed and is associated with a relatively low incidence of side effects. Ezetimide prevents cholesterol absorption and is also associated with a low incidence of side effects.

Check With Your Doctor!

There are many drug interactions between cholesterol-reducing medications and other medications. Some of these interactions are innocuous, although others are potentially dangerous. This is why a physician should be involved in the monitoring of any cholesterol lowering medication!

There is concern that some lower-dose statins may be sold over the counter in the future. Because the statins can be associated with adverse effects when combined with other medications, the use of statins and other cholesterol-lowering medications should remain supervised by a physician.

Possible drug interactions with statins and other cholesterol reducing medications:

Statins:

Possible dangerous interactions with drugs used for AIDS treatment: protease inhibitors

Antibiotics: erythromycin, clarithromycin, itraconazole, diltiazem, verapamil

Warfarin administered concomitantly with statins may lead to an increased risk for bleeding. The bleeding times should be checked frequently. These two medications should be administered under the care of a physician.

The resins cholestyramine and colestipol can bind statins in the intestine and prevent their absorption. Consequently, statins should not be taken one hour before or within four hours after taking the above resins.

Fibric Acids:

Warfarin administered with fibric acids may cause elevated bleeding times. One's physician should monitor one's warfarin closely while using fibric acids due to an increased risk of bleeding.

Grapefruit juice may affect the metabolism of fibric acids and should be avoided because it affects the liver metabolism of cholesterol-reducing medications.

Niacin:

Niacin may be absorbed by cholestyramine and colestipol, which prevents its absorption in the intestine. Consequently, niacin would be rendered ineffective. Niacin should not be taken within one hour before taking one of these resins. In addition, it should not be taken within four hours after taking one of these resins.

Niacin may interfere with aspirin (clinical relevance unclear).

Niacin may interfere with certain blood pressure medications.

Niacin may interfere with diabetes medications, such as metformin, glyburide, glipizide, or insulin preparations. Blood sugar levels should be monitored while taking these medications.

Niacin may interfere with the absorption and efficacy of certain antibiotics such as tetracycline.

Ezetimide:

Few drug interactions at this point. Specific questions should be directed to one's physician.

Colesevelam:

Few interactions at this point

The Least You Need to Know

◆ Powerful medications are available that help to reduce cholesterol levels.

◆ The main goal in cholesterol reduction is to lower LDL to the lowest levels possible.

◆ LDL cholesterol reduction therapy should begin early and be aggressive.

◆ There are many drug interactions between cholesterol-reducing medications and other medications. Patients should see their doctors regularly.

Chapter 20

Herbs for Your Health

In This Chapter

- Understand the effects that herbs have on the body
- Learn about the link between herbs and cholesterol levels
- Know why doctors don't back herbal supplements as a means to improve cholesterol abnormalities
- Learn the possible risks of taking certain herbs

Although there have been few scientific studies that demonstrate that herbs play a role in cholesterol reduction (or reduction in atherosclerosis progression and risk of heart disease in people with elevated cholesterol), many herbs contain compounds that affect human metabolism. In theory, then, these compounds could affect cholesterol levels. Some of these substances have been isolated from plants and other organisms and are used for medicinal purposes by modern physicians. For the most part, however, doctors generally don't recommend herbs as a substitute for proven cholesterol-reducing medications.

Because so many people are interested in herbs and their potential health benefits, I wanted to discuss them in this chapter, so that you have all the relevant information you'll need to make an informed choice on this front.

Alfalfa

Alfalfa leaf originated in the Middle East and was later imported to the United States. Alfalfa has been shown to reduce plaque volume and decrease cholesterol levels in animals. Alfalfa may also have some effect on macrophages, which play a part in plaque rupture and heart attacks.

Cooling Down Inflammation

Macrophages, if you'll remember, are inflammatory cells that circulate in body tissues. Macrophages typically release potent chemicals when they come into contact with a foreign body or germ. Macrophages, along with other cells dumping chemicals in the area, are to blame for the redness, swelling, and soreness in an area of inflammation.

The Doctor Says

Macrophages respond (along with other cells and chemicals) to an area of inflammation, releasing chemicals to fight germs of foreign bodies; however, these chemicals may also lead to plaque rupture and clot formation. Alfalfa may work to reduce the inflammatory activity of macrophages.

Many of these chemicals are similar to bleach, because they kill germs or break down foreign material. These inflammatory chemicals attract more macrophages to the area.

This destructive oxidative process can occur on the inside of blood vessels slowly over the course of a lifetime. If this happens, it usually results in atherosclerosis, heart attacks, or strokes. These chemicals may cause plaques to become unstable or to fracture. When the plaques fracture, of course, a blood clot can form on top of the weakened area, leading to a heart attack, or the blood clot can be dislodged and travel to the brain, causing a stroke.

If alfalfa stabilizes macrophages by preventing them from releasing their powerful inflammatory chemicals, it may reduce heart attacks and strokes! The possibility of preventing heart attacks and strokes by eating alfalfa will require additional scientific research.

Saponins

Alfalfa also contains a steroid-like group of compounds called saponins, which have a foamy or soapy appearance. Saponins are found in beans and may have anticancer effects, and immune-boosting and cholesterol-reducing functions.

Saponins bind cholesterol in the intestine and prevent its reabsorption. consequently, saponins function much like bile acid sequestrants, as both bile acid sequestrants and saponins inhibit the reabsorption of cholesterol in the intestine and excrete it in the stool.

Healthy Heart Facts

Many plants contain chemicals that have been noted to have effects on human health. Digitalis is a type of chemical that is found in the foxglove plant. For over 200 years, digitalis has been used in various forms to treat a weak heart; it's still used today in a medication called digoxin. Digoxin helps alleviate symptoms in people with heart failure but does not have any true beneficial effects in terms of improving the lifespan of these patients. In high doses, digoxin is toxic and causes nausea, vomiting, yellow halos around lights, and heart-rhythm problems.

Capsicum

Capsicum, or capsaicin, is the major ingredient of chili peppers. This compound has been demonstrated to relieve pain and is an anti-inflammatory. (Surprising news about a substance that burns your mouth!)

How does capsicum work? It inhibits a substance called *platelet-activating factor (PAF)*, which is involved with platelet activation, clotting, and inflammation.

After a plaque ruptures, the most critical element that causes blood to clot and subsequently causes a deadly heart attack is the platelet. When an injured area on the inside of the blood vessel is detected, platelets attach themselves to the area. In doing so, they release inflammatory chemicals that can attract other platelets (along with other cells) to the area. Because the area is now quite crowded with sticky platelets and other cells and debris, a blood clot may form.

def•i•ni•tion

Platelets are small disc-like cells that float around in the blood; they are produced by the bone marrow. Platelets are smaller than other blood cells and float through the blood searching for an injured area. These cells release an inflammatory compound called **platelet-activating factor,** or **PAF**, which contributes to the formation of blood clots.

One of the critical elements that platelets release is called platelet-activating factor (PAF). PAF is highly inflammatory and is increased in areas of blood clot formation as well as in areas of infection. PAF activates platelets and triggers a large blood clot.

What's remarkable is that blood clotting and infection are characterized by the release of the same or similar compounds, such as PAF. The body responds to a cholesterol insult on the inside of blood vessels the same as if there is an infection!

Potential natural sources of chemicals that may work to decrease excessive PAF production may be helpful for heart disease, high cholesterol, and infection. If chili peppers or capsicum are a natural source of compounds that inhibit PAF, there may be potential health benefits of these foods for us to explore. So you may be able to eat your (chicken) taco and enjoy heart health!

Garlic

Garlic has been used for centuries for its myriad effects, such as improving heart health and its antibacterial properties. There are more than 100 compounds in garlic that may be useful. Like all plants, garlic has adapted from an evolutionary standpoint to ward off the fungi and animals that may consume it.

Allicin is believed to be the main component in garlic; this is a complex, unstable molecule that's formed when garlic cloves are crushed or cut. So it's interesting to note that allicin does not actually exist in garlic; it's created when an enzyme in that does exist in garlic (called allicinase) acts upon an amino acid in garlic, alliin. Allicin is rapidly transformed into other substances. One substance is called diallyl disulphide, which possibly has medicinal effects.

Allicin as an Irritant

It has been claimed that the purported health benefits of garlic are due to allicin; however, it's unlikely that allicin reaches the tissues in any significant amounts, since it's an unstable element that's rapidly broken down by the harsh chemicals found in the stomach and intestine. Even enteric-coated allicin tablets may bypass the stomach, but they can't bypass the intestine.

In addition, even if allicin were to reach the intestine, it's an oxidizer, and it would likely act as an irritant to the intestinal tract. In fact, allicin may cause burns when applied to the skin. Some people may have allergies to allicin. One more problem to note with garlic: it has some anticlotting effects that may be problematic during the time following an operation, when bleeding is a concern. (So if you're taking garlic on a regular basis and you're scheduled for an operation in the near future, let your doctor know!)

The Doctor Says

One serious potential side effect of garlic is that its storage at room temperature in oil can lead to botulism. The combination of the chemicals in garlic and the oil can be a fertile ground for botulism bacteria. This is a potentially serious adverse effect of garlic. Consequently, garlic should never be stored at room temperature in oil.

Analysis of a Garlic Clove

One meta-analysis (a study that combines several studies into one) suggested that garlic might reduce LDL and total cholesterol. Another analysis of the larger studies in the previous meta-analysis suggested that there is no garlic/cholesterol-reduction connection. Some short-term studies suggested a cholesterol-reducing role for garlic, but longer-term studies failed to demonstrate a significant benefit. Although these studies may have been flawed in terms of methodology, there is little scientific literature to substantiate a true benefit from eating garlic.

Garlic has also been touted as a blood-pressure reducer. Similar to the cholesterol studies, there has been little scientific evidence showing that garlic is effective in reducing blood pressure.

Ginseng

Ginseng comes from the root of the ginseng plant and has been the subject of many types of health claims for nearly 7,000 years. The root can live for nearly 100 years and is native to Japan, North Korea, China and also can be found in parts of North America. Ginseng is thought to enhance …

◆ Energy.

◆ Memory.

◆ Immune system.

Ginseng is also thought to be a general panacea, as it's believed by East Asian cultures to optimize the body's overall functioning.

Ginseng has been studied for its possible anti-inflammatory benefits. It contains glycosides, or steroid-like substances called ginsenonides, which can potentially have anti-inflammatory activity. Ginseng also contains saponins, which, you'll recall from our discussion about alfalfa, may also be anti-inflammatory and may also have anti-PAF-like activity similar to other compounds that contain saponins.

Ginseng may affect *cytokines*, which are inflammatory substances released by cells when they are stimulated to mount a response to an infectious attack. Cytokines are also released by cells involved in atherosclerosis; during this process, cytokines attract other cells toward plaque to help in its formation and also in its disruption.

def•i•ni•tion

Cytokines are inflammatory substances released by cells when fighting infection. Cytokines also play a part in the development of atherosclerosis. Ginseng is thought to have an anti-cytokine effect.

There may be compounds in ginseng that have anti-cytokine activity. If these compounds have anti-cytokine activity, they may be anti-inflammatory and have a role in fighting atherosclerosis.

Turmeric

Turmeric is a plant found in India and is an important herb in ayurveda, or Indian medicine. Turmeric contains a compound called curcumin, which is believed to have anti-inflammatory activity. It's believed that an oil contained in turmeric produces its anti-inflammatory benefits. Although there is no evidence that turmeric reduces cholesterol levels, its anti-inflammatory activity may have beneficial effects on the progression of atherosclerosis.

Healthy Heart Facts

Turmeric is a plant and a member of the ginger family. A spice is made from the stalks that grow from the root. Turmeric grows in India, China, and Indonesia. This spice has a yellow color and can be found in curry and yellow mustard.

In the 1970s, it was discovered that turmeric contains a substance called curcuminoids. There were several studies that suggested that there may be anticancer and heart-disease benefits related to curcuminoids.

Other Herbs to Know About

After you start investigating herbs for medicinal use, you'll find that there are plenty to choose from! Some are safe; others are toxic and should be avoided. Below is a list of common herbs and the data that either supports or refutes their use. Except where noted, the efficacy of these herbs has not been proven; I have also made note of products that should not be taken!

As a word of caution, you should know that many herbs interact with medications administered by medical doctors and may lead to toxicity of the internal organs! Some of these herbs may also interfere with the metabolism of medications and lead to adverse side effects. Patients should inform their doctors of herbal remedies that they are taking! Ideally, before taking any herbal supplement, you should *ask your doctor to review your prescription meds and any herbs you're considering using as supplements*, using a reference source like the Physician's Desk Reference for Alternative Therapies. Don't feel funny about asking your doctor to specifically check with this text. Most doctors in the U.S. don't regularly use or recommend herbs; in addition, some herbal supplements may be unregulated.

> **Healthy Heart Facts**
>
> Before you take any herb, it's vital for you to understand any potential interaction it may have with the medications you are already taking! There are many, many places to get the facts about any herbs you may be considering. Look for books about herbal remedies, do some research online, or talk to your doctor or pharmacist.

- **Andrographis.** Has been touted to avoid second heart attacks after angioplasty.

- **Aristolochic acid.** This product was initially promoted for weight loss. It is actually toxic to the kidneys and is carcinogenic. It should not be used.

- **Artichoke leaf extract or cynara.** May reduce cholesterol. In addition, it may be helpful as a digestive aid.

- **Astragalus.** Has been promoted as a treatment for heart disease. It is frequently combined with other herbs in traditional Chinese medicine. It also has the name huang qi.

> **Here's to Your Heart**
>
> In the future, isolation of certain herbal compounds may reduce cholesterol. However, at the present time, there is no substitute for the use of diet, exercise, and medication for cholesterol reduction and management.

- **Chamomile.** Has been used as a sedative or anxiolytic. There have been other claims to its efficacy as well.

- **Chaparral.** Has been promoted as a cancer cure. However, it is hepatotoxic (toxic to the liver) and should not be used.

- **Comfrey.** May cause liver cancer and should not be used. Topical exposure is also not recommended.

◆ **Cordyceps.** Has been touted to reduce blood pressure and LDL levels.

◆ **Dan shen.** Has been used to relax the blood vessels supplying blood to the heart.

◆ **Dong quai.** Has been recommended for postmenopausal symptoms, but is likely ineffective. It may increase bleeding risk for Coumadin, which is a blood thinner that is often used for individuals with certain heart conditions.

◆ **Echinacea.** Has been promoted for its benefits against upper respiratory tract infections.

◆ **Ginger.** Has been promoted for motion sickness. It has also been promoted for nausea and vomiting in other situations and circumstances, such as related to pregnancy and after surgery. Its efficacy is unclear, but may be effective. The efficacy for ginger for post-operative pain is unclear.

◆ **Ginkgo biloba.** Has been effective for dementia. It may be effective for claudication.

◆ **Ginseng.** Has been promoted for improvement in physical and psychomotor performance. It has also been recommended for immune function, post-menopausal hot flashes, and diabetes. It has not been shown to be effective for these other indications. Notably, the American College of Obstetrics and Gynecology specifically recommends against its use.

◆ **Hawthorn.** Has been used for heart disorders. It may have a beneficial effect for mild congestive heart failure.

◆ **Horse chestnut seed extract.** This product has been shown to be effective chronic venous insufficiency. This product is given as a capsule twice daily before meals.

◆ **Kava.** Believed to have anxiolytic or sedative properties. It is toxic to the liver and not recommended.

◆ **Kombucha tea or Manchurian or Kargasok tea.** This product should be avoided. It has no proven efficacy for any indication and may cause severe acidosis. The use of this product is absolutely not recommended.

◆ **Milk thistle.** May be effective for liver cirrhosis. Milk thistle may be consumed as an extract three times per day.

◆ **Reishi or shitake.** May also lower cholesterol levels.

◆ **Saint John's wort.** Used for mild depression and is effective. It may be ineffective for major depression. Saint John's wort is available as an extract. Saint John's wort interferes with the metabolism of many drugs due to effects on the liver.

◆ **Yohimbine HCL or yohimbine bark extract.** These two products are not interchangeable. Nonprescription yohimbine is promoted for impotence and as an aphrodisiac. Yohimbine bark is considered unsafe by the FDA.

The Least You Need to Know

◆ Herbs may have a role in cholesterol reduction.

◆ More scientific research needs to be done on the link between herbs and health.

◆ Some herbs can interact with medications or affect their absorption; tell your doctor about any herbs you're using.

◆ Because some herbs are considered toxic to the body, make sure to carefully research any supplement you're considering.

◆ At this time, herbs are not recommended as a substitute for a healthy diet or cholesterol-reducing medications.

Chapter 21

Supplements and Natural Remedies for Your Heart

In This Chapter

◆ Find out which plant produces a statin

◆ Learn which supplements might be beneficial for cholesterol levels

◆ Understand what natural therapies are capable of achieving

◆ Educate yourself about the possible drawbacks of natural supplements and therapies

Despite all our advances in modern medicine, heart-disease therapy has proven to be highly elusive. The best therapy is prevention. The best prevention is through cholesterol reduction and management. The best cholesterol reduction and management is achieved through diet, exercise, and certain medications; however, some natural remedies have also been used with varying degrees of success. We discuss some of them in this chapter.

Many supplements and natural remedies have been used as alternative therapies for heart disease. We talk about some of the more common products that are floating around out there as a means of giving you the latest medical findings on these products. As you'll see, most of them have shown no scientific proof that they work to lower cholesterol. Before taking any of these supplements, discuss their use with your doctor; he may have some different recommendations for you to follow!

Red Rice Yeast

Red rice yeast is derived from a yeast that grows on rice and has been used as a food and medicine in the Far East for thousands of years. It decreases total cholesterol, LDL, and triglycerides and elevates HDL.

Mother Nature Does It Again!

Red rice yeast produces a group of compounds called menacolins, which block a particular enzyme in the liver. By inhibiting this enzyme, the yeast causes the liver to produce less cholesterol. Consequently, the receptor on the surface of the liver cells remove more LDL from the blood for cholesterol use by the liver. One type of menacolin found in red rice yeast is called mevinolin, which is marketed as lovastatin. That's right—this natural product produces a class of the highly effective cholesterol-reducing drugs we discussed in Chapter 18!

What's remarkable about red rice yeast is that it produces a substance that has a powerful effect on animal biochemistry. The promise of red rice yeast is that other substances will be isolated from other plants that will improve the health of people.

Common Uses

Red yeast rice was first used in 800 C.E. It's still eaten and used today in Asian countries. Red rice yeast has been used for myriad problems, including these:

- Digestive problems
- Cancer
- Lung problems
- Wound treatment
- Bruises

You may be able to find red rice yeast in pill form; however, there has been debate in the legal and pharmaceutical communities as to whether red rice yeast is a drug or a dietary supplement. A U.S. court ruled that products sold as red rice yeast cannot be distributed without a prescription because red rice yeast contains a prescription drug, lovastatin. Furthermore, red rice yeast preparations are not standardized; as a result, there's no way to determine how much lovastatin you're ingesting. It's recommended that red rice yeast be abandoned in favor of prescription statins for cholesterol reduction.

> **Healthy Heart Facts**
>
> A derivative of red yeast powder has been produced that contains policosanols, a group of compounds that inhibit cholesterol formation. We'll talk more about these compounds later in this chapter.

Guggul Tree Resin

This substance has been used for several thousand years in India as part of ayurveda, or Indian medicine. Guggul tree resin contains a compound called guggulsterone. Studies have demonstrated that guggulsterone binds to a liver receptor; by interacting with this receptor, cholesterol synthesis is decreased by the liver. The effects of guggulsterone on the liver receptor were demonstrated in studies conducted at Baylor College of Medicine in Houston, Texas.

The role of guggulsterone in cholesterol lowering is not likely to be significant. Some studies have actually suggested that guggul tree resin can increase cholesterol. It's safer to follow traditional medicine's approach and use statins for cholesterol reduction.

> **Healthy Heart Facts**
>
> Practitioners of ayurveda have to get their guggul from somewhere! Guggul resin is derived from the guggul tree, which grows in arid regions of India, Bangladesh, and Pakistan. The resin is harvested from the tree from November through January by cutting into thee bark and allowing the resin to seep out. A typical guggul tree will produce up to one pound of resin per year.

Policosanol

Policosanol is derived from sugar-cane wax and is a combination of alcohols. It's available in pill form. The recommended dosage is 5 to 20 mg per day, and side effects include nausea, headache, and dizziness.

The effects on of policosanol on cholesterol include reduction of total cholesterol, LDL, and triglyceride, as well as elevation of HDL. Policosanol may be useful for people seeking an alternative to modern medicines, because policosanol is a plant-derived product.

The substance also affects LDL receptors and may affect the oxidation of LDL. Let's back up a step and talk about oxidation. LDL can become more dangerous to cell membranes by becoming oxidized. (We call this oxidant damage.) Oxidized LDL encourages cholesterol to deposit itself on the inside of blood vessels and also encourages the development of heart disease. Policosanol, meanwhile, is believed to play a role in blocking the detrimental oxidation of LDL. We'll get into oxidation in much more detail in Chapter 22.

> **Healthy Heart Facts**
>
> One study showed that policosanol was more effective in cholesterol reduction than one of the statins, fluvastatin!

Octacosanol

Octacosanol is one compound that forms policosanol and is its active ingredient; it's found on the blades of wheat plants and is also present in some vegetable oils, such as wheat germ oil.

Octacosanol has been used by body builders and athletes, as it has been claimed that it enhances physical performance. It has also been claimed that octacosanol can be used for Parkinson's disease, *although there is no valid data to substantiate this*. Octacosanol is administered as 1 to 8 mg by mouth per day in a capsule or tablet form. A dosage of 20 mg has been recommended as the maximum dose. However, it hasn't been shown to lower cholesterol in scientific tests. It's recommended that statins and approved medications and techniques be used to lower cholesterol instead of octacosanol.

Pantetheine

Because pantetheine plays a major role in metabolism, it has been marketed as an energy booster. Some studies have demonstrated that pantetheine can reduce total cholesterol and triglyceride and increase HDL. Pantetheine may also affect the fluidity of platelet membranes and the production of a substance called thromboxane A2. Let me break this down, so that it's a little clearer:

◆ Platelet fluidity involves platelets' ability to clump and cause blood clots.

◆ Thromboxane A2 is a major platelet agonist, which means that it stimulates platelets to clump and releases other substances that are inflammatory and to produce blood clots. It's kind of like the bad seed, egging on the formation blood clots.

The actual mechanism of action of pantetheine is not known, though we do know that it's a vitamin B5. It may not hurt to add pantetheine to your daily regimen, but it shouldn't be used in place of cholesterol-lowering medications and treatments (such as diet, exercise, and medication) that have been proven to be effective in scientific studies.

Curcumin

Curcumin is the main component of turmeric, a spice obtained from a plant. It may have anti-inflammatory activity by reducing the activity of platelet-activating factor (PAF), which we talked about in detail in Chapter 20. Because PAF has a powerful role in the inflammation associated with heart disease, blood clotting, and infection, curcumin may have beneficial effects on the progression of atherosclerosis.

The Doctor Says

LDL deposited in the arteries creates an inflammatory situation which, for one thing, encourages more cholesterol to join the party, so to speak. This inflammation also encourages the development of a clot in the blood vessel, which can lead to a heart attack or stroke. Anti-inflammatory substances can reduce this risk!

Beta-Sitosterol

Beta-sitosterol is a member of a group of compounds called plant sterols and stanols. These are substances that prevent absorption of cholesterol in the intestine, though their mechanism of action (or how they work, exactly) isn't completely understood.

Here's what we do know about these compounds: consuming two grams a day of plant sterols or stanols will reduce LDL by about 25 percent! In turn, this will achieve about a 25 percent reduction in cardiovascular mortality, as for every 1 percent reduction in LDL, there is a 2 to 3 percent reduction in cardiovascular mortality. Plant sterols and stanols are not widely available.

Psyllium

Psyllium is a medicinal plant that has been used for thousands of years in Asia, Europe and Africa. Herbal medicine uses the seeds of the plant for its purported benefits.

The Doctor Says _____

Because psyllium may reduce blood sugar in diabetics, taking it may necessitate an alteration in insulin doses. If you're a diabetic taking psyllium, make sure to tell your doctor about it!

Chinese and ayurvedic physicians have used psyllium to treat various ailments including digestive and respiratory problems. In addition, psyllium can lower blood sugar and cholesterol levels by preventing its absorption into the bloodstream. Because psyllium is the main ingredient of laxatives, it should be used cautiously by individuals who take prescription drugs, as its effects may reduce their absorption.

Licorice Extract

Licorice root has been used for thousands of years as a treatment for the following ailments, among many others:

- ◆ Respiratory disorders
- ◆ Digestive disorders
- ◆ Skin disorders
- ◆ Neurologic disorders
- ◆ Immune disorders

The Doctor Says _____

In concentrated amounts, glycyrrhizinic acid can potentially cause electrolyte abnormalities and elevated blood pressure. So although it may be tempting, keep your licorice consumption to a moderate amount!

Such amazing effects from something that most kids (and adults) consider a treat!

The major component of licorice is glycyrrhizinic acid, which has a steroid-like effect. There may also be other useful components of licorice; we know, for example, that licorice without the glycyrrhizinic acid is thought to heal ulcers.

There does not seem to be much of an effect of licorice on the bloodstream or blood vessels. At this time, there is no direct scientific evidence linking licorice with reduced cholesterol levels or the prevention of the progression of atherosclerosis or heart disease.

Natural Therapies

The consequences of elevated cholesterol, of course, may include life-threatening heart disease. Many natural therapies have been advocated to have benefit. For example, Coenzyme Q has been used as a therapy for heart muscle disease. Magnesium may or may not benefit heart attack victims. Chelation therapy and homocysteine reduction have had mixed reviews in the treatment of elevated cholesterol. We'll talk about each of these natural therapies in this section.

Coenzyme Q

Coenzyme Q is a component of the cell membrane. It participates in the transfer of electrons from one *intermediate* to another in cell metabolism. Coenzyme Q participates in this process and is also an antioxidant within cells. It can be taken in a pill form and has been produced and has been marketed commercially as a remedy for various heart illnesses, ranging from heart muscle pain (called angina) to heart failure.

def•i•ni•tion

As all cells use oxygen to acquire energy from glucose and other substrates, various **intermediates** are created during cell metabolism that participate in the harnessing of energy. The energy is transferred in the form of electrons from one intermediate to another.

Although there are substantial claims that Coenzyme Q is a highly effective therapy for heart disease, there is no objective data in the medical literature that Coenzyme Q has any use for heart-disease management. The scientific studies to date have actually yielded powerful evidence suggesting that the therapy is ineffective.

Magnesium

Magnesium is an element that's required for use by key enzymes in the human body. This mineral has had widespread claims of effectiveness in the management of heart disease. Huge, scientifically conducted rigorous studies, on the other hand, have revealed no benefit for magnesium in the management of heart disease unless there is a clear deficiency of magnesium, which is rare but can happen with certain cancer treatments and also with the use of water pills.

For many years there was a debate both inside and outside the traditional scientific community on the possible benefits of magnesium for heart disease. (In other words, both doctors and natural healers were talking about this.) Some of the early studies with magnesium suggested that it could stabilize platelets and the membranes of the heart cells, decreasing the likelihood of life-threatening heart-rhythm disturbances during and immediately after a heart attack.

Many physicians used to routinely prescribe magnesium to their patients who came to the emergency room with a heart attack. It was generally believed that magnesium

The Doctor Says

Magnesium has many potential positive beneficial effects on the heart, the blood vessels, and on various cells, but as I've already said, there's no scientific proof that it works.

was not harmful; plus, magnesium deficiencies are difficult to detect, so for all these doctors knew, heart-attack victims were suffering from a magnesium deficiencies. And because some life-threatening cardiac arrhythmias are treated with magnesium, it certainly seemed like a logical conclusion to make. In addition, magnesium supplementation is relatively inexpensive, which makes it accessible in almost every hospital setting.

The combination of all of these factors created ample opportunity to market and recommend magnesium as a treatment for heart disease, and magnesium deficiency as a cause of heart disease. It took many years to lay the magnesium controversy to rest. Even today, there are still critics within the cardiac community who point out deficiencies in the studies that were conducted and who recommend a reexamination of magnesium.

Chelation Therapy

Chelation therapy is the intravenous infusion of a substance called ethylenediaminetetraacetic acid, or EDTA for short. This substance is used to remove heavy metals, such as lead, from the body during episodes of heavy-metal poisoning or toxicity. The heavy metal binds to the EDTA and is removed from the body in the urine.

This theory has been carried over into the realm of heart disease, the speculation being that removal of calcium would regress atherosclerosis. The theory is flawed because calcium removal and reduction in the incidence of plaque rupture are unrelated.

Healthy Heart Facts

Patient involvement in therapies that are outside of mainstream medicine (such as chelation therapy) may be harmful because patients are deprived of therapies that have been proven to be effective and to save lives. This is one reason studies of natural therapies are necessary.

Plaques that typically rupture are often noncalcified and are soft, allowing them to break easily. To date, the theory is unproven. The American Heart Association does not recommend chelation therapy as a form of heart disease treatment.

To resolve the chelation controversy, two branches of the National Institutes of Health—the National Center for Alternative Medicine and the National Heart, Lung, and Blood Institute—are conducting a study called the Trial to Assess Chelation Therapy, or TACT. Results are expected in 2007.

Homocysteine Reduction

For many years, it was believed that the reduction of homocysteine, an amino acid produced by the body, was associated with a reduced incidence of heart disease. This link between homocysteine and heart disease initially developed when it was noted that an enzyme deficiency involved with the breakdown of homocysteine in the body led to dramatic elevations of homocysteine. This in turn caused a marked increase in the incidence of heart disease. Recently, less dramatic elevations in homocysteine have also been associated with an increased incidence of heart disease.

Based upon these association studies, it's theorized that the treatment of elevated levels of homocysteine would lead to a reduced incidence of heart disease. Because the therapy for elevated homocysteine is relatively innocuous, consisting of vitamins B_6 and B_{12} and folic acid, it's been suggested that starting treatment for this condition even without some conclusive scientific evidence to support the treatment may be harmless and may be associated with possible benefit.

However, a recent large study determined that therapy for elevated homocysteine with the goal of homocysteine reduction was not associated with any benefit to the heart. As a result, reduction of homocysteine may no longer be a therapeutic goal.

The Least You Need to Know

♦ Before you begin taking any supplement for cholesterol reduction or heart health, speak with your doctor!

♦ Red rice yeast actually contains lovastatin, which is a statin.

♦ Most supplements have not been shown to improve cholesterol levels.

♦ Chelation therapy has not been shown to remove calcium from the body.

♦ Currently, there are no natural therapies that can take the place of a health diet, exercise, and prescription cholesterol-lowering meds.

Chapter 22

Antioxidants and the Heart

In This Chapter

- ◆ Learn about the normal, toxic substances that are a by-product of metabolism

- ◆ Get the full story on oxidants and the damage they can cause in the body

- ◆ Understand how LDL can become even more damaging in the presence of oxidants

- ◆ Know what antioxidants do to help protect the body against oxidative damage

- ◆ Find the best sources of antioxidants

Toxic substances in the human body are unavoidable, at least when they're the by-products of metabolism. Our body breaks down, or oxidizes, substances (such as food) into their most basic components, and not all of these components are healthy or beneficial to the body. Fortunately, the body has various methods of neutralizing these products of oxidation, or oxidants. The compounds that the body produces to counteract these compounds are called antioxidants.

We've talked a bit about oxidation in some of the earlier chapters; in this chapter, we go further into the details of antioxidants and what they can do to your cardiovascular health.

What Antioxidants Can Do for Heart Health

We hear about antioxidants all the time. They've become a common selling point of vitamin manufacturers who claim that their products provide antioxidants in concentrations high enough to be good for our health. What does this mean, though? We know that oxidation is a normal, albeit damaging, effect of metabolism, but what does any of this have to do with the heart?

Some of the oxidative damage that happens during metabolism occurs in the membranes of cells that line blood vessels (endothelial cells); some of the damage occurs in the cells that are involved with inflammation and blood clotting (platelets). Some of the damaging substances, or *oxidants*, are called *free radicals*. These are charged metabolic *intermediates* that are toxic to various cell components and can cause damage over time.

def•i•ni•tion

Antioxidants are compounds that occur naturally in the body. They help to prevent damage caused by charged compounds called **oxidants,** which are also a natural by-product of the metabolic process. One type of damaging oxidants are called **free radicals.**

Intermediates are substances created during cell metabolism. They participate in harnessing energy and passing it from one intermediate to the next in the form of electrons.

In theory, *antioxidants* prevent inflammatory damage and clotting, which, you'll recall, creates a dangerous situation inside the blood vessels by increasing the risk of heart attack and stroke. This all starts with the breakdown, or metabolism, of the food we eat.

In the next section, we go through the oxidation process step by step to understand what happens in the body and what kind of damage may be done. But don't worry—we come back to antioxidants later in the chapter.

How Oxidation Does Its Damage

The foods that we eat are complex molecules. By complex, I mean that food is made up of molecules that have energy stored in the bonds between carbon atoms. This energy is released from these bonds during metabolism.

This next part is a bit complicated, so I'm going to break it down into small, bite-sized pieces of information:

◆ Part of this process of metabolism produces intermediates, compounds that have extra electrons and a negative charge.

◆ This negative charge on the intermediates can damage other molecules that are also charged on their surfaces, like the lipids that make up all cell membranes.

◆ Because all the components of a cell are contained in a tiny package bound by a membrane, the many structures inside the cell can be damaged by the intermediates.

◆ These intermediates are especially dangerous when they are produced in the area of cholesterol plaque. They are highly inflammatory and can promote the rupture of plaque.

Now, the good news is that the body has defense mechanisms that are capable of neutralizing these charged molecules. The defense system is also built into the metabolism of the cells and destroys the charged molecules as soon as they are produced. We'll talk about this process a bit later in this chapter.

Oxidants and Plaque

As damaging as oxidative compounds can be, the human body can harness the dangerous potential of intermediates and have it perform a useful function, like destroying invading bacteria. When you use bleach to disinfect your home, the bleach destroys the cell membranes of bacteria. These charged compounds act in the same way toward bacteria in the body. Cells that are capable of destroying bacteria contain packages of oxidizing, or bleaching, substances that destroy bacteria when they come into contact with them.

Here's the problem, though: cells that form plaque and cause them to rupture are similar to the cells that destroy bacteria. When cholesterol accumulates on the inside of the blood vessels, it attracts inflammatory cells to the area deposit bleaching substances on the inside of the blood vessel. Obviously, this is a harmful situation.

Here's to Your Heart

It's unlikely that cholesterol plaque can be entirely avoided; however, a healthy diet and cholesterol-reducing medications will most likely reduce the chances of attracting inflammatory cells to participate in the rupture process and the depositing of bleaching oxidants.

It's important to understand that the bleaching or oxidizing substances are not the culprits. They're part of the cells in the body that fight infection; they're just doing their job! This controlled oxidation is a necessary part of life. The best way to avoid this type of oxidant injury to the blood vessels is to not have the cholesterol plaque in the first place!

Oxidized LDL

Atherosclerosis, or the narrowing of the arteries caused by cholesterol deposits, is a chronic condition; it tends to be worse in people who have many risk factors. (You'll recall that we discussed risk factors for cardiovascular disease in Chapter 5.) Oxidants can make this bad situation even worse.

def•i•ni•tion

The amount of plaque that occupies a three-dimensional space is called **plaque volume.**

The higher a person's total cholesterol, LDL, and triglycerides, the greater the likelihood of significant plaque accumulation, or *plaque volume*, on the inside of the blood vessels.

Plaque volume is increased in people who have a combination of the following risk factors:

- High total cholesterol
- High LDL
- Low HDL
- High triglycerides
- Tobacco smoking

- High blood pressure
- Diabetes
- Advanced age
- Obesity

The Doctor Says

The best way to minimize oxidative LDL is to treat the risk factors that are responsible for the excessive LDL levels and the LDL oxidation in the first place. Risk-factor treatment includes smoking cessation, dietary therapy, weight loss, exercise, and medications.

A person can survive many years, even to old age, with atherosclerosis. However, people die because of plaque rupture or the development of a fissure within the soft plaque that triggers inflammation and clotting. Most heart attack or plaque rupture triggers are not known. However, we do know that oxidized LDL is a powerful trigger for plaque rupture.

What makes LDL oxidized? The LDL floating around the blood stream is taken up by macrophages, or inflammatory cells, in the cholesterol plaque. If there is excessive oxidative stress in the body due to poor diet, tobacco smoking, diabetes, and other risk factors, the LDL is more likely to become oxidized. The oxidized LDL is consumed by the macrophages, which then initiate a powerful inflammatory response.

You already know that macrophages play a role in plaque rupture. In short, macrophages that have consumed oxidized LDL can cause plaque rupture much more easily than macrophages that have consumed nonoxidized LDL.

Oxidized Mornings

There are periods of heightened vulnerability where cardiovascular events are concerned, or times when plaques are more likely to rupture. For example, doctors have noted that in the general population, plaque rupture tends to happen after infections and after flu season.

Astonishingly, it's also been known for many years that heart attacks, strokes, chest pain, and elevations of blood pressure often occur before awakening. The actual event of waking up in the morning is incredibly stressful for the body. (It's not just your imagination!) During this time, there's usually a surge of sympathetic activity, which, if you recall from Chapter 17, makes the body's various systems work harder.

> **Healthy Heart Facts**
>
> Because the period of awakening can lead to so many cardiovascular events, doctors often prescribe heart medications that will prevent this early morning surge in cardiovascular events.

Even more interestingly, studies have shown that changing your sleep patterns to awake at night only moves the surge in cardiovascular events. In other words, sleeping through the early morning surge doesn't prevent cardiovascular events; it only delays the surge to when you do wake up! Controlling the risk factors associated with elevated LDL helps to prevent oxidized LDL from playing a role in plaque rupture. Correcting both conditions may help to decrease these periods of vulnerability upon awakening.

Antioxidants to the Rescue! (Maybe!)

Cholesterol deposits are really part of an inflammatory disease. As cholesterol levels rise, more cholesterol is deposited on the inside of blood vessels. Before a heart attack, there is a sudden increase in inflammation in the area near of the plaque that is about to rupture. You could say that the inflammation encourages the rupture.

You've read how powerful oxidants in the region of the plaque are involved with the triggering of a heart attack. Antioxidants may quell the local inflammation and decrease the likelihood that the plaque will rupture. But…this is only a theory.

> **Healthy Heart Facts**
>
> Statins help to stabilize plaque, reducing its likelihood of rupture. Other agents that stabilize plaque and prevent rupture include aspirin and some medications (such as beta-blockers or ACE-inhibitors) given to patients after a heart attack. These medications can also be taken by individuals who are at risk for heart attack.

The field of antioxidants is controversial. There is strong evidence that oxidation is involved with plaque rupture and subsequent heart attack. However, although a diet rich in antioxidants is associated with a reduced likelihood of heart attack, there is no definitive proof that consuming antioxidants will decrease the likelihood of plaque rupture.

At this time, the most effective way to lessen the risk of oxidative-related events, including inflammation, is to consume a healthy diet and exercise regularly. In addition, using cholesterol-reducing medications will reduce the amount of plaque available to rupture, which in turn will decrease the risk of heart attack and stroke.

Sources of Antioxidants

The best sources of antioxidants are healthy foods. The foods that we eat supply the body with the necessary products to manufacture antioxidants at a cellular level. Taking antioxidants in a pill or tablet is not likely to provide any antioxidant boost at a cellular level.

Foods Versus Supplements

Many studies have been conducted investigating dietary supplements versus an adequate diet. The prevailing opinion, based upon all of these studies, is that there is no supplement that replaces a healthy diet!

Most compounds that alter human cell metabolism—and, subsequently, oxidation—are not known. Of the compounds that have been discovered, isolated, or extracted from plant food, few of them are understood completely in terms of their effects upon human metabolism. Because many degenerative diseases including heart disease and cancer are characterized by oxidative damage, it's in your best interest to consume a diet that is likely to reduce oxidant damage.

To minimize oxidative damage, it's wise to eat a diet that includes lots of these good foods:

- ◆ Fruits
- ◆ Vegetables
- ◆ Grains
- ◆ Legumes
- ◆ Fish

Here's to Your Heart

As with foods containing vitamins and minerals, antioxidants need to be consumed in food form to achieve benefit. Other compounds contained in healthy foods likely affect the way foods metabolize in the body, which in turn affects the oxidation process.

The Paleolithic diet, for example, will reduce cholesterol and reduce the amount of plaque on the inside of the blood vessels. By reducing the plaque for the oxidizing substances to act on, the effects of oxidation (such as plaque rupture and heart attack) will be reduced. In addition, the need for antioxidants drops when blood vessels are healthy and cholesterol-free.

Antioxidant Drips?

Although we can infuse certain medications to help ease some of the symptoms or risk factors involved with heart attacks and strokes, at this time, there is no way we can increase levels of antioxidants in the vicinity of a plaque that is about to rupture.

Although medical scientists may discover antioxidant drugs in the future, the best current mechanism to prevent oxidation-related atherosclerosis and heart attack is to lower cholesterol. Lowering cholesterol may be achieved through consumption of a Paleolithic diet, regular aerobic exercise, and the use of proven cholesterol-reducing drugs, such as statins. (These approaches to cholesterol reduction will also help reduce blood pressure, reduce insulin resistance, and reduce overweight and obesity.)

Healthy Heart Facts

It has never been demonstrated that a person can supplement the diet with antioxidants and decrease the amount of oxidizing substances released by the inflammatory cells or reduce the effects of oxidants. The benefits of antioxidants appear to come from a healthy diet.

Antioxidants and Statin Drugs

In Chapter 18, we discussed how statins may have multiple, or pleiotropic effects. In other words, statins may protect against heart disease through mechanisms unrelated to LDL reduction. Although the issue of pleiotropic effects is somewhat controversial among physicians, it's believed that some of the statins' far-reaching positive effects may be related to an antioxidant effect that statins have on the blood vessels and inflammatory and clotting cells.

Beyond the possible antioxidant effects of statins and the possible adverse interaction between vitamin E and statins (which we'll talk about in the next section), antioxidants should be consumed as part of a healthy diet. When combined in this fashion, dietary antioxidants may have beneficial effects in conjunction with statins.

Dangerous Interactions

Various substances that have been presumed to be antioxidative have been tested in human studies. The results are mixed. Vitamin E, for example, is presumed to have antioxidant qualities, and large studies have been done to determine the role of vitamin E in preventing oxidative damage. The consensus of these studies is that vitamin E provides no benefit as an antioxidant. In fact, some studies have shown that taking certain antioxidants with other medicines can actually be harmful when used in conjunction with other medicines! In one study, vitamin E was associated with increased cardiovascular risk when combined with statins.

Because the role of statins in heart disease prevention, management, and reduction of cholesterol abnormalities is indisputable, statins should not be withheld in favor of vitamin E, no matter what its supposed antioxidant qualities may be!

The Least You Need to Know

- ◆ Oxidation is a normal part of the metabolic process.
- ◆ Oxidants can cause damage to cells; free radicals are one type of oxidants.
- ◆ Inflammation and clotting can be caused by oxidation.
- ◆ LDL can become oxidized, which makes a bad situation in the arteries even worse!
- ◆ Antioxidants help to stop or minimize the damage oxidants can cause.

Chapter 23

On the Horizon

In This Chapter

- ◆ Read about new cholesterol drug therapies in development
- ◆ Learn about drugs that may help to get rid of plaque in a hurry
- ◆ Understand how treatment of one disease may also help to improve other conditions
- ◆ Become educated in genetic defects
- ◆ Share in our hopes for better heart health in the future

Over the past few years, there has been a trend to increase the dosage of statins in patients who have high cholesterol as well as use combination therapy when appropriate. In addition, the Adult Treatment Panel of the National Cholesterol Education Program (NCEP/ATP III)of the National Heart, Lung and Blood Institute has also suggested that cholesterol target numbers be reduced. Research is now focusing on more powerful statins and other new drugs that target cholesterol abnormalities through different mechanisms.

In this chapter, we talk about some of the drugs under development that may be successful in raising HDL levels, and we also talk about therapies that seem to go beyond the scope of cholesterol reduction, but bring their results right back to the health of your heart.

New Drugs Under Development

One example of a new cholesterol-altering therapy has been the development of drugs that specifically target HDL. It's possible that the role of HDL may have been underestimated, a situation that may have been partially due to the difficulty in changing its levels. HDL rises minimally with various interventions including diet, exercise, and medications. Although it'd been pointed out that relatively minor elevations in HDL may be associated with relatively large health benefits, future innovations in raising HDL may yield dramatic elevations and give us even greater health benefits.

HDL and Plaque Volume

A drug that is currently being considered for HDL elevation is called torcetpamib. This is an intravenous medication that can achieve rapid HDL elevations. Because HDL removes plaque from arteries, rapid elevations may elicit a rapid removal of plaque from the inside of the blood vessels.

Why is this such big news? A drug that acutely raises HDL and reduces the amount of plaque on the inside of an artery immediately after a heart attack may be useful. To fully understand the reasons why this may be so, we need to first discuss LDL and plaque volume.

def•i•ni•tion

The amount of space the plaque occupies in three-dimensional space is called **plaque volume.** Plaque volume is measured with a thin ultrasound probe that is passed down the inside of a blood vessel.

When statins are administered to lower LDL during a heart attack immediately after admission to the hospital, they have some benefit. However, the studies that have been performed over the past 15 years or so have demonstrated a very small reduction in the size of the cholesterol plaque when statins are given to a person with heart disease. The reduction in plaque size, or *plaque volume*, takes at least a few months, often longer.

Despite a very small reduction in the thickness of the cholesterol plaque noted on the angiogram when statins were given to people with heart disease and high cholesterol, there was a marked reduction in heart attacks and heart disease related death. Statins may change the composition of the plaque, not its size. Essentially, the statins made the plaque more stable and less prone to rupture. This is good, but cardiologists want medications that do even more! Read on.

Keeping Our Fingers Crossed ...

Statins achieve dramatic benefits in terms of reducing heart disease–related death in spite of the fact that they have a minimal effect on the size of the plaque. So just think of the benefits of using a medication that not only has an effect on lipids—such as raising HDL—but that also dramatically reduces the size of the plaque! A medication like this should, in theory, have a profound effect on the reduction in cardiovascular events such as heart attack and stroke!

Currently, studies are demonstrating dramatic and rapid reductions in cholesterol-laden plaque (as assessed by intravascular ultrasound). Potentially, many years of cholesterol deposits could be removed rapidly. The implications are tremendous. Consequently, there's a lot excitement in the medical community about drugs that increase HDL and dramatically and quickly reduce plaque size. It may be premature, however, to conclude that cholesterol-laden plaque may be removed so quickly. More research is needed, but doctors are excited.

More Statins, Stat!

In addition to HDL-raising, plaque-reducing drugs such as torcetpamib, more powerful statins are being investigated that may achieve greater reductions in LDL. There's also an increasing emphasis being placed on combining various drugs that are used to affect multiple subfractions. Newer drugs are being developed to interact with different cholesterol pathways to decrease LDL, raise HDL, and decrease triglycerides.

The Doctor Says

Many people worry about taking a statin, thinking that the risk of liver and muscle toxicity outweighs the benefits of the drug. In reality, the risk of not taking a statin when you have elevated cholesterol and other risk factors for heart disease is often greater than the uncommon side effects of statins, which are usually recognized and corrected early on with regular monitoring for liver and muscle enzyme abnormalities.

Lose Weight, Feel Great!

Along with new drugs targeting HDL elevation, there are likely to be new drugs to treat the constellation of abnormalities called metabolic syndrome, a group of disorders linked by several factors, such as:

- Poor diet
- Lack of exercise
- High blood pressure
- Abnormal cholesterol levels
- Insulin resistance

The person who suffers from metabolic syndrome is overweight and has high cholesterol. Insulin resistance may be the central abnormality linking the various components of the disorder. A new medication called rimonabant has been demonstrated to achieve significant weight loss in overweight individuals by blocking a receptor called the cannabinoid receptor; in doing so, a person experiences early satiety, or the feeling of being full without overeating.

Drugs Doing Double Duty

Often, abnormal cholesterol levels coexist with elevated blood pressure, obesity, and early diabetes as we see in the case of someone afflicted with metabolic syndrome. And often, these diseases are treated the same way because interestingly, treatment of one disease such as diabetes may affect other diseases, such as cholesterol abnormalities.

> **Healthy Heart Facts**
>
> Rimonabant's weight-loss effects are achieved without the side effects of other weight loss medications, which raise adrenaline levels and affect the serotonin system, resulting in heart valve disorders and pulmonary hypertension, a deadly disorder associated with elevation of the pressure in the lungs.

There is evidence, for example, that newer drugs called triazolidines, or TZDs, may improve cholesterol and diabetes simultaneously by working on a receptor that is common to both diseases, called the PPAR-alpha. Basically, there's overlap at a basic cellular and biochemical level between the two diseases. Because TZDs work at this common level, they're able to improve both conditions. Examples of TZDs that are commonly prescribed include pioglitazone and rosiglitazone. There is currently investigation into whether these drugs can also be used to prevent heart disease.

Overweight Mice and Your Heart

Interestingly, in mice, there is actually a gene for obesity called leptin, a protein that prevents mice from getting full and stop eating. The role of leptin in human obesity is still being investigated, but with any luck, one day scientists will be able to say with certainty whether this gene or another one can be altered to help obese people lose weight. Because obesity is linked with high cholesterol and heart disease, such a discovery could also potentially improve cardiovascular health for overweight individuals.

Awareness Is the Key!

In general, the latest trend in cholesterol management is that it's becoming more aggressive. There is a growing emphasis on earlier intervention, lower LDL numbers, and higher HDL levels. In addition to the medications being developed for the purpose of raising HDL levels, new drugs are also being developed to target smoking cessation and metabolic syndrome.

Public awareness of the dangers of elevated cholesterol is increasing. A major hurdle in preventing heart attack and stroke will be overcoming societal inertia. It may be quite difficult to motivate people to change eating habits and activity levels. So although doctors have piles of scientific research and new therapies in our corner, these changes in societal thinking and behavior pattern may be more difficult to achieve than new drug development and improved cholesterol targets.

> **Healthy Heart Facts**
>
> Often, scientists will set out to create a drug that helps one condition and find that it also helps another. Rimonabant is used to help people lose weight, but it's also been shown to improve cholesterol and glycemic levels, and help with smoking cessation. Rimonabant is still in clinical trials.

Gene Therapy

The current degenerative diseases that have plagued humans in the twentieth and twenty-first centuries are a combination of genetics and environment. Many serious health conditions have a genetic component to them. Diseases that are thought to have at least a partial familial link include these:

> **The Doctor Says**
>
> There are lots of ethical issues surrounding gene therapy, such as insurability and discrimination. (Will someone with a 'defective' gene be able to get health insurance? Will employers be able to demand employees seek medical attention for predetermined risks?) So as remarkable as some of these studies are, we must be careful to temper their findings with compassion and common sense.

- ◆ Diabetes
- ◆ Obesity
- ◆ Heart disease

The good news is that the genetic components to these conditions are now being unraveled. *Gene therapy* could isolated defective genes and correct them, resulting in amazing and dramatic benefits to an individual's health!

Single Gene Mutations

Some genetic diseases are due to *single gene mutations* that are well understood because of we can isolate the one defective gene. Some diseases and illnesses are due to multiple mutations in a single gene. Two examples of a single gene defect that causes illness are sickle cell anemia or Marfan syndrome. These illnesses are fairly well understood genetically.

By contrast, illnesses and syndromes such as high cholesterol, high blood pressure, type 2 diabetes, and obesity are likely due to the effects of many genes, most of which are unknown. The goals of gene therapy include changing the course of these illnesses by manipulating the genes.

def•i•ni•tion

Genes are long DNA molecules that are located on chromosomes. The chromosomes are located in the center of all human cells. There are 23 pairs of human chromosomes in the nucleus (or central command center) of each and every human cell. **Gene therapy** seeks to isolate one defective gene and change it, thus alleviating any illness it has been causing.

A **single gene mutation** is a defect in one gene that causes illness. High cholesterol may be caused—at least in some instances—by a mutation in several genes, making it a more difficult genetic condition to understand. One such genetic elevated cholesterol condition is called **familial hypercholesterolemia**.

Genetics and Cholesterol

One type of severe cholesterol disorder, termed *familial hypercholesterolemia*, is caused by a genetic defect or mutation wherein the receptor on the liver cells that binds to LDL is completely absent. Because LDL can't be removed from the circulation by the liver LDL receptor, it deposits itself elsewhere in the body—and what a horror this turns out to be for an individual's health.

In familial hypercholesterolemia, LDL deposits as plaque throughout the arteries in the body starting at a very young age. Individuals with this disorder have been known to have heart attacks in infancy, childhood, and adolescence. Their LDL levels may rise into the hundreds or thousands!

Healthy Heart Facts

There are some other disorders that are characterized by LDL receptor deficiencies or abnormalities that are less severe than familial hypercholesterolemia. These individuals may also have very high LDL levels, but not as high as those who have a complete absence of the LDL receptor.

In recent years, there has been interest in replacing the absent or aberrant gene responsible for familial hypercholesterolemia with a functional gene. The technique is still experimental, but doctors are keeping a hopeful eye on the data.

Keeping Your Options (and Blood Vessels) Open

Although reimplanting deficient or dysfunctional genes will be remarkable, the technology responsible for successful reimplantation is still in its infancy. However, some incredible strides are being made at this time, and again, doctors are keeping a watchful eye on the future of this field of medicine.

One such advance is in the field of angioplasty. After someone has an angioplasty to reopen a narrowed or closed blood vessel, there is a very high rate of reocclusion of the vessel. Typically, reocclusion, or *restenosis*, occurs in about one third of the individuals who have this procedure, depending on the blood vessel involved. (Some blood vessels experience an even higher rate of restenosis!) Recent advances have decreased this restenosis rate significantly by utilizing metallic implants, or stents, within the artery.

def•i•ni•tion

When an artery that has been opened by angioplasty closes up again, we refer to that process as **restenosis**. Gene therapy scientists are currently researching methods by which to deliver a gene into a blood vessel to prevent this renarrowing.

The restenosis that occurs within a stent is due to a new form of atherosclerosis. The stent actually allows for the inside of the blood vessel to grow and reocclude the artery. Gene therapy researchers are looking for ways to deliver genes to the inside of the blood vessels using balloons and stents as platforms. These genes could, theoretically, turn off the growth process of the inside of the blood vessels. The genes can be delivered in manmade capsules that have a fatty coating or may be injected into the blood vessel cells using viruses that have been genetically modified to be incapable of causing disease!

Vascular Endothelial Growth Factor (VEGF)

After a heart attack occurs, the cells dependent upon the blood vessel die and are replaced by nonliving scar. Sometimes, the blood vessels nearby develop sprouts or collaterals to bypass the closed off vessels and provide circulation to the dying or dead

def•i•ni•tion

Vascular endothelial growth factor (VEGF) is a gene responsible for the sprouting of new blood vessels. It's also responsible for allowing some cancers to metastasize. Researchers are currently looking for a way to harness VEGF's properties to allow new blood vessel growth around the scar tissue left by a heart attack.

areas. The blood vessel cells manufacture a substance called *vascular endothelial growth factor (VEGF)*, which stimulates the growth of baby blood vessel sprouts.

Incredibly, this substance, although important for the heart, can also cause blood vessels to form in tumors and allow for their early spread or metastasis. As a result, VEGF has good and bad properties in the body. Researchers are experimenting with ways to deliver VEGF to the heart using angioplasty equipment to deliver the gene that codes for VEGF directly into the heart blood-vessel cells.

This remarkable technology is experimental, but holds a promise of possibly being able to either turn on good genes or turn off bad genes.

Although the blood vessel regrowth experiment is exciting, researchers have already discovered that this isn't as easy as simply plugging VEGF into a blood vessel and watching new vessels come to life. One needs to administer many growth factors in addition to VEGF (which is a growth factor itself), either as the compound itself or as the gene that codes for the compound.

The Least You Need to Know

- There are aggressive therapies in the pipeline for improving cholesterol abnormalities.

- Many of the new therapies are focused on increasing HDL and dramatically reducing LDL.

- Some of the new medications seek to quickly reduce plaque volume, resulting in a lowered risk of heart attack and stroke.

- Various drugs are being investigated that may improve the multiple components of the metabolic syndrome.

- Genetic therapies for improving cholesterol levels and heart health are still a long way off.

Part 5

Dr. Klapper's Step-by-Step Plan for Losing Cholesterol Points

Want to know what I tell my own patients? It's all contained in Part 5. Along with advice for dietary modifications, quitting smoking, and exercise tips, you'll also read that not all cholesterol-reducing meds are created equally. I'll let you in on the medications I prefer to use for my patients and explain why I may choose one drug over another.

Please note that this is a guide to help you better understand the decisions your own physician may make as far as your care is concerned, not a guide for self-treatment. Educated patients who follow their doctors' advice are more likely to succeed in their health goals!

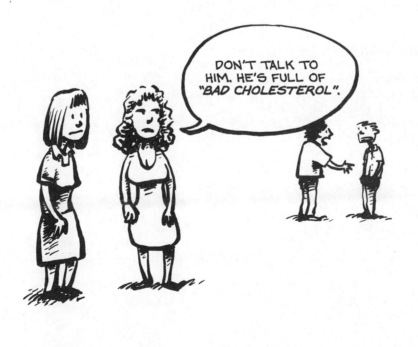

24

Dr. Klapper's Plan for Healthier Living

In This Chapter

- ◆ Know why you should have your cholesterol checked early and regularly
- ◆ Set a good example for the kids
- ◆ Accept exercise as part of every day
- ◆ Decide that you're going to quit smoking
- ◆ Understand the medications available for smokers who want to quit

Cholesterol reduction is based upon three major approaches, which form a three-pronged attack. The basic components of the three-pronged attack include diet, exercise, and medication. I'll talk about my specific recommendations for diet and exercise as they relate to cholesterol reduction in this chapter; in the following chapter, I'll talk more about medications for lowering cholesterol. There are also other lifestyle modifications that are necessary for cholesterol reduction and heart health, such as quitting smoking. Effective ways to kick your nicotine habit will be discussed in this chapter.

As you apply this guide to your own life, I can't overemphasize how important it is for you to seek the advice of your own physician! Your doctor needs to take your health and cholesterol levels into consideration, so that the two of you can discuss how to come up with a plan that works best for you. A doctor is the best person to formulate an overall risk-stratification profile and provide necessary follow-up. Moreover, many people may underestimate the severity of their risk factor profile. Someone with a normal total cholesterol level may have abnormal cholesterol subfractions (high LDL, low HDL) that place them at elevated risk.

Remember: this guide is to be used in conjunction with your doctor's advice, not in place of it!

> **Here's to Your Heart**
>
> By lowering your cholesterol, you will reduce your risk for heart disease, stroke, and other illnesses. We know that by reducing cholesterol, blood vessel health is improved. And improvement in blood vessel health leads to a reduction of illnesses of all sorts!

Starting Early

Although the formal guidelines promoted by various health agencies suggest an initial cholesterol panel at age 20 (with a follow-up within five years if normal and a repeat with subfractionation if abnormal), I recommend a more intense and aggressive pursuit. My advice is more consistent with the evolving school of thought within the medical community that cholesterol target numbers should be reduced and interventions to lower those numbers should be more aggressive.

In this section, we talk about ways to help start the entire family on a healthy-living regimen.

> **The Doctor Says**
>
> The United States is in the throes of an epidemic of obesity and diabetes. A significant proportion of this morbidity and mortality is determined at a young age.

Early Prevention, Early Treatment

I recommend an adolescent risk-factor assessment that includes cholesterol screening. The reason I recommend earlier intervention at younger ages is that coronary artery disease due to cholesterol abnormalities begins at a young age. In addition, dietary and exercise patterns are often determined at a young age, and some of the damage caused by poor dietary choices and lack of exercise are likely irreversible. Addressing high cholesterol at an early age gives your child plenty of time to *prevent* cardiovascular disease!

Intervention for lowering cholesterol needs to begin at a young age, but you can't treat a condition that hasn't been diagnosed. Consequently, I recommend early screening of children for risk factors that may lead to heart disease later in life. Cholesterol measurements are particularly important at a young age, especially in children who are overweight or obese and who have a family history of heart disease and other risk factors.

Lead the Way, Mom and Dad!

I recommend that parents discuss diet and exercise with their children. The discussion of proper diet and regular exercise with children serves not only to improve the health of children but also to improve the health of adults, because teaching is a learning experience.

The same thought that goes into choosing foods for the adults in the household should enter the decision-making process when parents teach their children how to eat. It's particularly important for parent to teach children to avoid foods that are high in simple sugars and dangerous fats, such as junk foods and fast foods. Other tips for modifying your children's diets include the following:

◆ Replace sugar-laden carbonated beverages with water, juice with no sugar added, or low-fat milk. It's important for adults to read juice labels, as many juices frequently are low in actual fruit juice and high in added sugar.

◆ Use fat-free or skim milk products. Milk products are good sources of protein and calcium but are sometimes high in fat. (Reduced fat or 1-percent milk may be better than whole milk but still contains much fat.)

◆ Ice cream should be minimized and may best be offered to children as a treat perhaps once per week. Similarly, ice pops that are high in sugar should be avoided. It's easy enough to make ice pops at home from fruit juice.

◆ Kids can eat a Paleolithic diet, too! Push those fruits, vegetables, low-fat meats, and whole grains! They're low in fat and high in nutrients, which are essential for growing bodies.

Lifting the Remote Is Not Exercise

In addition, it's important for parents to encourage children to exercise regularly and to choose physical activities over a sedentary lifestyle. Children should look for ways to join in physical activities and avoid watching excessive television and playing video games, especially while eating junk foods.

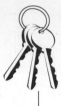

Here's to Your Heart

In addition to its benefits to the heart and its prevention of the development of obesity, exercise also helps to prevents diabetes. It has been estimated that one out of three children born in the year 2000 are destined to develop diabetes! In view of this frightening statistic, it becomes even more relevant to educate children on the importance of healthy eating patterns and daily exercise at a young age.

It's not difficult to get kids to exercise. Examples of activities that may be performed with children include …

◆ Walking to school.

◆ Jumping rope.

◆ Using stairs instead of elevators.

◆ Participating in outdoor activities, such as baseball, basketball, and games incorporating running and jumping.

◆ Enrolling in organized athletics, such as martial arts, basketball, softball, swimming, or whatever activity your child most enjoys.

In addition, children should accompany their parents to the market when it's time for the weekly grocery shopping. This helps to demonstrate and reinforce the healthy choices made by the parent while shopping.

The Doctor Says

Because smoking increases the risk of heart disease, it's important for you to send a clear message to your kids: *Don't start smoking!* It's much easier to never smoke at all than to kick a nicotine habit later in life. Stand firm on this issue, even if you're a smoker yourself. And if you *do* smoke, I've got another great reason for you to quit: Second-hand smoke is also a significant risk factor for heart disease, so your children may be suffering the consequences of your smoking even if they never light up themselves.

Exercise Program

One of the three prongs in the attack against high cholesterol is daily aerobic exercise. This book has discussed several exercise programs. In beginning an exercise program, you should determine the goals you have in mind. If your main goal is to reduce cholesterol through aerobic exercise, you should choose an aerobic program. If your goal is to increase muscle strength and mass, a weight-training or resistance program is ideal.

Including Exercise in Your Daily Routine

Aerobic forms of exercise include walking, fast-paced walking, jogging, running, or swimming. You can increase the level of exercise as your fitness level increases by increasing the amount of time you spend exercising and by increasing the pace of the activity. Before you increase the intensity of exercise training, you should realize that exercising to achieve cholesterol-reducing benefits and to improve your general health does not require the performance of high-intensity activity. Studies have revealed that moderate activity is sufficient to achieve the cardiovascular benefits that most people are looking for.

In terms of cholesterol management and improvement of cardiovascular and general health, exercise has to become a way of life. Exercise is a continuous choice between activities. These choices are similar to the choices you make in the supermarket about which foods to purchase. People who want to lower their cholesterol and improve their health will choose physical activity over nonphysical activity whenever the choice presents itself. For example, a health-minded individual may choose to …

♦ Use the stairs instead of the elevator or escalator.

♦ Walk to work instead of driving.

♦ Go for a walk instead of watching television.

♦ Perform several minutes of jumping rope in the morning instead of relaxing with a newspaper.

> **Healthy Heart Facts**
>
> Typically, for improvement of fitness level and for cholesterol reduction, an exercise program that is primarily aerobic is most useful; however, it's important to recognize that programs that incorporate resistance training can be quite aerobic if performed properly. I recommend a combination of aerobic and strength training for maximum benefits.

Do you see where this is going? You have to learn to recognize opportunities as they present themselves during a the day to modify your lifestyle and take it from being sedentary to active. In addition, during both work and leisure time, you should seek to maximize activity as opposed to inactivity.

It's important to emphasize that a sudden shift from an inactive, sedentary lifestyle to completely active and nonsedentary is probably not going to happen, and is also probably not the best way to ensure that you'll stick to a new, more active lifestyle. Rather, try to alter your thinking and gradually change the your lifestyle.

Here's to Your Heart

An active lifestyle should be combined with a Paleolithic diet! Cavemen and primitive man didn't have television and video games for entertainment. A caveman didn't sit at a computer terminal, talk on a telephone, or drive an automobile on a freeway to a desk job. The caveman also didn't have high cholesterol and heart disease. Mimicking this lifestyle (to a certain degree—no need for you to actually move into a cave) is likely to yield health benefits for you in the twenty-first century!

Two Workouts in One

Typically, for improvement of a person's fitness level and for cholesterol reduction, an exercise program that's primarily aerobic is most useful, but it's important to recognize that programs that incorporate resistance training can be quite aerobic if performed properly. For example, if you were doing some weight training, you could reduce the length of the rest period between sets and increase the number of repetitions per set. These two modifications tend to increase heart rate and achieve greater aerobic benefits.

It's also important to keep in mind that most forms of exercise use aerobic exercise as well as resistance exercise. For example, training on a heavy punching bag is highly aerobic yet incorporates resistance training as well, because hitting a heavy bag requires the use of considerable muscle strength.

Check In for a Checkup

Before you begin any exercise routine, you should have a basic assessment of your fitness level done by your physician. This can usually be performed without having to resort to testing or other sophisticated objective analyses of levels of fitness, but, if need be, your doctor can use certain tests to evaluate your level of fitness. Poor fitness is an extremely powerful prognosticator of mortality. In some studies, the most powerful risk for heart disease mortality is one's level of exercise tolerance.

One way to determine your fitness level is to undergo a *cardiopulmonary stress test*. Because the heart and lungs work together, this technology assesses the function of both systems together. Doctors (including myself) recommend this technology only for people who have specific symptoms, such as decreased exercise tolerance or shortness of breath. However, even in these situations, it's unusual to undergo a cardiopulmonary stress test. If your physician suspects underlying heart disease, a treadmill test using a continuous electrocardiogram (a monitor of the heart's electrical activity while one is exercising on a treadmill) may provide useful information. If your doctor suspects a lung problem, he may choose to perform lung test.

def•i•ni•tion

A **cardiopulmonary stress test** measures for both the heart and lungs and is usually only performed for individuals when a physician has difficulty determining which component— the heart or the lungs—is responsible for adverse symptoms. This test can measure the amount of oxygen that is consumed by the body. This measurement, called a VO2, gives a rough estimate of someone's level of fitness.

Quit Smoking

Tobacco cessation is a key component to cholesterol reduction. Although cholesterol is not reduced by tobacco cessation and although tobacco smoking does not elevate cholesterol, tobacco smoking is associated with increased amounts of plaque on the inside of the blood vessels. Because the amount of plaque on the inside of the blood vessels is associated with a greater risk of plaque rupture and subsequent heart attack and stroke, smoking increases risk for these adverse events.

Diet + Exercise + Meds + *No Smoking!*

I've talked a lot about the three-pronged approach to lowering cholesterol. Here's something you should consider: all the effort you put into making these cholesterol-reducing, health-improving lifestyle modifications will be nullified by tobacco smoking. Period. There's no getting around that. Tobacco smoking is such a powerful risk factor that it will render all other health-related interventions nearly worthless.

This is not to dissuade anyone from exercising and eating a healthy diet. Not exercising, eating an unhealthy diet, and smoking tobacco are associated with markedly increased risk for adverse outcome including stroke heart attacks, cancer, and premature death.

It's (Cold) Turkey Day!

Tobacco cessation is best done cold turkey, or all at once. Reducing the number of cigarettes smoked per day is ineffective. In addition, switching to low-tar cigarettes won't do you any good. These are no less dangerous that regular cigarettes.

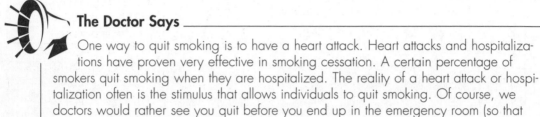

The Doctor Says

One way to quit smoking is to have a heart attack. Heart attacks and hospitalizations have proven very effective in smoking cessation. A certain percentage of smokers quit smoking when they are hospitalized. The reality of a heart attack or hospitalization often is the stimulus that allows individuals to quit smoking. Of course, we doctors would rather see you quit before you end up in the emergency room (so that you don't end up there at all!)

Sometimes, the advice given by a physician or other health care provider is especially effective at helping smokers to kick their habit. Studies have shown that when doctors advise their patients to quit smoking, their patients usually listen. This kind of intervention by a physician may be as simple as a gentle reminder to a patient to quit smoking, but its effects are often indelible.

Smoking Stoppage Steps

Smoking cessation consists of all the steps required for any bad habit to be broken. However, quitting smoking may be much more difficult than, say, doing away with your habit of cursing like a sailor, for several reasons.

First, smoking is a learned behavior. People incorporate smoking into their basic adapting and coping skills. For smoking cessation to be successful, individuals often need to find other outlets or other ways to cope. Think about this: people often incorporate smoking into their basic relationship skills. To quit smoking, smokers often need to learn to interact with other people without relying on tobacco. Consider how smokers will smoke after dinner or during a conversation or will ask for a cigarette to initiate a conversation with someone. Furthermore, consider how the use of cigarettes relieves anxieties and provides a pleasurable experience during various forms of anxiety-arousing situations. The psychological and physical experience of cigarette is self-rewarding and reinforcing.

The first step involved in quitting a smoking habit is to understand that tobacco is detrimental to your health. Most people in today's society are familiar with the dangers of tobacco smoking. Everyone reads (or at least hears about) the Surgeon General's report. We're bombarded with media attention and information regarding the dangers of smoking. People watch their friends and family die from heart attacks and cancer. There are very few people who do not understand the dangers of smoking or who have not been inundated with the antismoking propaganda. In addition, there are very few people who are not aware that their smoking habit is also harmful to nonsmokers. Consequently, most people have already achieved step one. (That was easy!)

Step two is making the decision to quit smoking. This is a big step, because although you may know in the back of your mind that you should quit, and you may even be thinking that you will quit, actually deciding to quit is an entirely different thought process. When you've made this decision, it may a good time for you to talk to your doctor. When a health professional becomes involved with an individual who has decided to quit, there is a greater chance for success.

Here's to Your Heart

Smokers should understand that they are likely to experience one or more setbacks or relapses after quitting. Relapses should not be viewed as failures but simply as steps involved in the process of tobacco cessation.

Healthy Heart Facts

Don't feel like a failure if you've quit and gone back to smoking! Many people will quit smoking after experiencing a heart attack but will start up again at some point. These individuals may receive smoking-cessation intervention and be successful at quitting, because they've already demonstrated that they can do it!

The third step is setting a quit date and choosing a realistic date to quit. The date to quit should not be a long way in the future, as that may indicate that you're really not ready to quit. (Six months from tomorrow you're going to light your very last cigarette? I'm willing to bet you're going to forget about it—maybe on purpose, maybe not.) A good quit date may be a birthday (yours or a loved one's), an anniversary, or the date of a previous heart attack.

After your quit date has arrived, go cold turkey. Various medications are available that may facilitate the process of quitting. We'll talk about them at the end of this chapter.

Try, Try Again

Smokers who have quit may experience many relapses. Try not to be too discouraged. *Try again.* You're not alone if you do experience a relapse. Oftentimes, smokers may require several attempts to quit smoking, but they are successful at becoming smoke-free in the long run.

Smokers may need to engage in various forms of therapy to quit smoking. Therapy is important in that smoking served a coping role and provided psychological and physically reinforcement. The void left by smoking may need to be replaced with other coping mechanisms. Often, smokers will replace smoking with overeating. In the smoking-cessation circumstance, overeating is not discouraged, because it is easier to shed several pounds than it is to quit smoking. In addition, smoking is more dangerous than being overweight, so weight gain is not considered an adverse effect of smoking cessation from a health standpoint.

Medications for Smoking Cessation

Many smokers find it very hard to quit. Fortunately, we're living in an age where there are several medications available to help make the process easier. I've listed these prescriptions in this section for your easy reference:

- **Buproprion.** Available by prescription. Take 150 mg once or twice per day. Start with 150 mg once per day × 3 days and increase to twice per day for 7 to 12 weeks. The maximum dose is 150 mg twice per day. Side effects include seizures in less than 1 percent.

- **Nicotine gum.** Take by gradually tapering to one piece every one to two hours for six weeks, one piece every two to four hours for three weeks, and then one piece every four to eight hours for three weeks. The maximum dose is 30 pieces per day of 2 mg or 2 pieces per day of 4 mg.

- **Nicotine inhalation system.** Use 6 to 16 cartridges per day for 12 weeks. Oral inhaler contains 10 mg per cartridge. 4 mg of nicotine is delivered per cartridge. A box contains 42 cartridges.

- **Nicotine lozenge.** For those individuals who smoke less than 30 minutes from waking, use 4 mg lozenge. Others should take 2 mg lozenge: take 1 to 2 lozenges every 1 to 2 hrs × 6 weeks; then take every 2 to 4 hours during weeks 7 through 9; and then take every 4 to 8 hours in weeks 10 through 12. The length of therapy is 12 weeks.

- **Nicotine nasal spray.** Take one to two doses each hour. Each dose is two sprays, one in each nostril. Each spray has 0.5 mg of nicotine. The minimum recommended dosage is 8 doses per day with a maximum of 40 doses per day.

- **Nicotine patches.** Apply one patch (14 to 22 mg) per day. Taper the dose of the patch after six weeks. Individuals should not smoke when the patch is applied.

The Least You Need to Know

- Having cholesterol panels checked while you're still feeling healthy is a great way to prevent disease.

- Parents need to set a good example for their children by instituting a low-fat diet in the home.

- Regular exercise has been shown to lower LDL and raise HDL levels.

- Although smoking doesn't cause elevated cholesterol levels, it does encourage plaque deposition on the blood vessel walls.

25

Dr. Klapper's Prescription for Lowering Cholesterol

In This Chapter

- ◆ See why statins are my first choice of drug therapy
- ◆ Understand my reasons for prescribing other cholesterol-reducing meds
- ◆ Learn how I target multiple cholesterol abnormalities
- ◆ Know how to monitor for enzymes and other adverse symptoms

In addition to the tips I've laid out in Chapter 24, medication very often plays an integral role in lowering cholesterol. In this chapter, I'll give you the same recommendations concerning cholesterol-reducing medications that I give to my own patients, along with my rationale for using them, so that you can make an informed decision about your own care when you speak with your doctor.

All cholesterol-reducing drugs come with the risk of side effects. The potential for side effects, though slight in many cases (especially with the use of statins), increases with the use of multiple cholesterol-reducing medications. Your doctor needs to be aware of the medications you're taking so that he can monitor your overall health and keep an eye on enzyme levels that may be affected by the use of various medications.

Statins

Although much of the benefit of the statins is achieved with low-to-intermediate doses, I attempt to maximize dosage, as studies have revealed that higher dosages are associated with greater benefits. (The greater the LDL reduction, the better for the patient.) As long as individuals can tolerate the statin dosage, I use this therapy as the main attack against cholesterol.

Furthermore, although there is a difference in opinion in the medical community—two schools of thought, one advocating the pleiotropic effects of statins (those that go beyond lowering LDL), the other minimizing them—I prefer to maximize the statin dosage in case the school of authors who ascribe to the pleiotropic effects is correct.

Starting Statins

I usually start with simvastatin or atorvastatin as my main statin choices for patients. The mortality data for simvastatin is particularly robust, so I typically will choose this medication first. Atorvastatin is usually my second choice because the mortality data is not available. I may choose another agent such as pravastatin if I believe I will need to add a fibric acid. In this situation, pravastatin use is less likely to lead to statin toxicity when combined with a fibric acid.

The Doctor Says

Simvastatin is usually my first or second choice for statins. It is potent and may be used up to 80 mg per day. Simvastatin has a strong database and rigorous clinical trials support its use.

The reason I choose statins over other medications is because they very likely reduce mortality based upon the LDL hypothesis, which states that LDL is detrimental and that lower is better.

I typically don't make major changes in statin choices after therapy has begun. If an individual's prescription plan covers one statin and not the other, I may continue a statin I would not otherwise have chosen, because I prefer that patients take a statin rather than discontinue the medication because they cannot afford it.

Atorvastatin

I often use atorvastatin because it's associated with dramatic reductions in LDL, total cholesterol, and triglyceride. It's also associated with relatively marked elevations in HDL. Like all statins, atorvastatin has been demonstrated to have greater benefits in those patients at highest risk. In other words, diabetics and individuals with multiple risk factors or known heart disease will benefit the most from atorvastatin.

> **Healthy Heart Facts**
>
> The figures speak for themselves: atorvastatin is associated with 29 percent to 45 percent reductions in total cholesterol and 39 percent to 60 percent reductions in LDL.

Depending on how high the LDL is and how high the risk, I start patients out with a 10 mg dose of atorvastatin and increase to 40 mg by mouth per day. The highest dose is 80 mg per day. For individuals with very high LDL levels and increased risk, I'll start with a higher dose.

I usually obtain a liver and muscle enzyme panel at two weeks, then at six weeks, three months, and six months. There are three enzymes that I pay particular close attention to. The first two enzymes are liver enzymes called AST and ALT. To assess for any muscle damage, I also check a muscle enzyme called CK.

 The Doctor Says

Sometimes, the muscle enzyme CK can be elevated from taking certain medications or from a strenuous workout, but it can also result from a heart attack. If I'm concerned about a heart attack, I immediately hospitalize the individual and perform other diagnostic tests that clearly indicate whether there's been a heart attack. People with high cholesterol and other risk factors can have a silent high attack, which presents without chest discomfort but which is associated with damage to heart muscle that is detectable on a blood test.

I also prefer to monitor liver and muscle enzyme elevations frequently because patients usually have other medical problems, such as hypertension and diabetes that may require follow-up blood work if they are taking any medications that affect their electrolytes. These diseases necessitate closer monitoring, especially if individuals are taking multiple medications. In these cases, I usually draw electrolytes along with liver and muscle enzymes.

Listed below are a few other checks I do when prescribing atorvastatin:

◆ A cholesterol panel at two to six weeks, depending on the situation.

◆ If an individual has had a recent heart attack and his or her LDL is elevated, I'll usually check cholesterol earlier, perhaps two to four weeks after starting atorvastatin, because I want to be sure I'm not underdosing it.

◆ Finally, I question the patient about unusual muscle aches or soreness that isn't clearly linked with some activity or injury. If unusual muscle pain is present, I will stop the atorvastatin and check a CK.

If muscle pain is an issue, I may also do another enzyme test (an aldolase level) to detect muscle damage. Uncommonly, muscle breakdown can occur without elevations of muscle enzymes, which is something to keep in mind, because muscle aches and pains and soreness out of the ordinary will typically indicate that this is an issue.

Pravastatin and Fluvastatin

Pravastatin is my third-choice statin. I use pravastatin frequently because there is a strong base of data to support its use. Pravastatin also has a long history of use and is prescribed from 40 to 80 mg by mouth per day.

I don't often use fluvastatin, because it's less potent than say, simvastatin. That means that I typically have to prescribe a much higher dose to achieve the same LDL reductions that another statin could achieve with lower dosages. I will continue someone on this drug if a patient's insurance plan covers it and not other statin choice. I usually won't discontinue it unless there are adverse effects.

Sometimes, I'll switch to a more powerful statin such as atorvastatin and simvastatin, especially if the patient has markedly elevated LDL and multiple risk factors. Switching medications is usually a clinical judgment call made after incorporating the individual's lipid subfractions and risk factors. For fluvastatin, I use the same monitoring frequency as I described above for atorvastatin.

Lovastatin and Rosuvastatin

Lovastatin can be administered from 20 to 80 mg per day, and there is an extended-release version available. I usually choose atorvastatin and simvastatin over lovastatin unless an individual is already on the medication and is tolerating it well or his insurance plan covers lovastatin.

Rosuvastatin is prescribed from 10 mg to 40 mg by mouth per day. It is a new medication and quite potent. There is a new combination drug on the market that combines ezetimide and rosuvastatin.

The Doctor Says

The reason that cardiologists prefer one statin to another is usually based on clinical trials and their results. All statins reduce LDL; all cardiologists believe that the LDL theory (LDL reduction translates into lowered risk of cardiovascular disease) is true. We want to lower LDL, obviously, so we usually will use the statins that have the best scientific data indicating reduced mortality rates.

Bile Acid Sequestrants

The bile acid sequestrants are older medications. They used to be primary therapy for LDL reduction until the statins arrived on the market in the early to mid-1990s and proved their efficacy at reducing cardiovascular events. The bile acid sequestrants, meanwhile, have not been demonstrated to reduce overall mortality.

Colesevelam is the only widely used bile acid sequestrant. I add this to the statins as secondary therapy when LDL remains high. Another choice is ezetimide. Both medications have little chance of significant side effects. For patients with high triglycerides, I try to avoid colesevelam, because bile acid sequestrants may elevate triglycerides. In general, I try to maximize the statin dosage and add ezetimide to drive down the LDL.

The benefit to utilizing ezetimide is that it reduces LDL and triglyceride, and elevates HDL without any serious side effects. The favorable side effect profile is related to the fact that ezetimide is not absorbed. Another benefit of ezetimide is that it can be used in combination with a statin.

Healthy Heart Facts

Cholestyramine powder and colestipol are other types of bile acid sequestrants that are not commonly used. In general, the older bile acid sequestrants were associated with gastrointestinal side effects that made taking them unpleasant. Because the statins do such a remarkable job of lowering cholesterol without side effects, these older medications are nowadays most often left on the pharmacy shelves.

Fibric Acids

The fibric acids are useful for lowering elevated triglycerides and raising low HDL. This type of situation is frequently seen in people with insulin resistance or metabolic syndrome. Fibric acids can be combined with statins when there are lipid abnormalities besides elevated LDL.

I recommend a fibric acid for low HDL or elevated triglyceride. If patients have low HDL levels after beginning a statin and maximizing the dose, I recommend adding gemfibrozil or fenofibrate. The gemfibrozil data is especially convincing. One important study showed that cardiovascular events were reduced in people who had low HDL if when they were taking gemfibrozil.

Healthy Heart Facts

In large scientific trials in the 1980s, the fibric acids demonstrated a reduction in nonfatal heart attacks but no reduced overall mortality patients had been on these medications for many years. Another study recently looked at the use of fibric acids in diabetics. The findings were similar to those of the previous study: heart attacks were reduced but overall mortality was not.

When adding a fibric acid to a statin, I try to use pravastatin as the statin of choice because it's less likely to lead to toxicity when a fibric acid is added. Gemfibrozil, in particular, is associated with a greater risk of toxicity when combined with statins other than pravastatin. Gemfibrozil may also be preferable for individuals at higher risk and with lower HDL. Low HDL is a powerful risk factor and should be treated with agents that have demonstrated cardiovascular benefit.

When concerned about side effects, I tend to use fenofibrate because it's associated with less toxicity when combined with a statin. I will add colesevelam to a statin for additional LDL reduction. Your doctor should follow your triglyceride levels when using bile acid sequestrants, because they may increase triglycerides.

Niacin

The data for niacin in terms of reducing cardiovascular events is not as strong as it is for statins. Although niacin has profoundly beneficial effects on triglycerides and HDL, there is limited data on its effects on hard endpoints, such as heart attack and stroke. In addition, niacin is associated with many side effects, such as the following:

◆ Increased blood sugar, which can worsen a diabetic state

◆ Increased uric acid (possibly resulting in gout in those predisposed to the condition)

◆ Flushing of the face

The best way to avoid the flushing associated with niacin is to increase the dose slowly and to administer aspirin, acetaminophen, or ibuprofen 30 minutes before taking niacin.

Typically, niacin is my last choice for combination therapy because it has a greater side-effect profile. The evidence in its favor primarily came from study that used niacin in combination therapy with statins, and not as an isolated compound. I will use niacin for LDL reduction, triglyceride reduction, and HDL elevation, but prefer to try fibric acids first.

Niacin Dosages

When I do advise patients to take niacin, I recommend the following forms and dosages:

◆ **Immediate-release niacin.** Take 50 to 100 mg by mouth two to three times per day with meals, increasing the dose slowly. The usual maintenance dose is 1.5 to 3.0 mg per day. The maximum is 6 mg by mouth per day.

◆ **Extended-release niacin.** Start with 500 mg by mouth before bed. Increase slowly, monthly, as needed, to two grams per day. The maximum dose is two grams per day. The extended release formulations may have greater liver toxicity.

Again, the best way to avoid the flushing associated with niacin use is to increase the dose slowly and to take aspirin, acetaminophen, or ibuprofen 30 minutes prior to taking niacin.

Lovastatin and Niacin

These two medications are available as a combination. There's a trend in treatment of blood pressure, cholesterol, and diabetes to use multiple agents that target multiple pathways. This kind of treatment is convenient for the patient and increases compliance, because there are fewer pills to take. The downside of combination therapy is that it comes with increased risk for side effects and drug interactions with other drugs, because more medications are being taken.

Follow Up and Retesting

Individuals taking statins or other cholesterol-reducing medications should follow up with their doctors for ongoing monitoring and retesting. Patients should have their lipid panels (with subfraction analysis) evaluated on a frequent basis while taking statins, fibric acid, and niacin.

Healthy Heart Facts

The goal of cholesterol-reduction therapy is to drive the LDL to the lowest possible level. The greater the patient's risk, the greater the LDL-reduction goal. So even if LDL levels are within the normal range, the values should be driven even lower if someone has risk factors for heart disease.

I follow liver function tests and muscle enzymes frequently. In addition, I recommend questioning patients about muscle tenderness or soreness. Patients frequently have several disorders going on at the same time. Many disorders may have similar root causes, so treating one condition will frequently treat the others, as well. While drawing blood for liver and muscle enzyme analysis, it's helpful to check electrolytes, kidney function, and other variables that are important to the follow up and treatment of other disorders that may also be present.

Targeting Multiple Cholesterol Issues

One person can have problems in every area of his or her cholesterol subfractions: elevated LDL, elevated triglyceride, and low HDL. This, unfortunately, is a common situation. Patients with multiple cholesterol problems will require multiple medications to target the multiple subfraction abnormalities.

The Doctor Says

Some people may have underlying liver disease. If I have any concern about an individual's liver, I will likely refer the patient to a liver specialist for advice on whether the patient can receive cholesterol-lowering medication.

Typically, in treating patients with multiple cholesterol abnormalities, I start with LDL-lowering therapy, usually a statin. After starting the statin, I recheck the lipid panel four to six weeks later to reassess the levels. If the LDL remains elevated, I'll increase the dose of statin or add ezetimide. Sometimes, I'll add ezetimide instead of increasing the statin dose if I'm worried about the patient's liver. I rarely use a statin plus a fibric acid plus niacin, but some high-risk patients may require all three.

The decision to begin a statin or other medication in a patient with multiple medical problems and possible drug interactions needs to be made on an individualized basis using sound clinical judgment. This judgment incorporates the individual's risk for heart disease plus his or her risk for adverse effects when taking statins or other lipid-lowering medications.

Parting Shots

Fish oil, as you know, has been shown to improve blood-vessel health. There are several fish oil preparations. I suggest about two to four grams per day in divided doses, usually two to three times per day. Fish oil capsules should contain a mixture of DHA and EPA. One side effect of fish oil is fishy burps.

Finally, patients with elevated cholesterol frequently receive aspirin at 81 mg per day, unless there are contraindications. This recommendation needs to be individualized and decided for each patient by a physician using his or her best clinical judgment.

The Least You Need to Know

- ◆ Statins are usually the first course of drug therapy for elevated cholesterol.
- ◆ Doctors usually choose a statin based on how well it's done in clinical trials.
- ◆ Drug therapy for reducing cholesterol should be accompanied by a doctor's monitoring of a patient's enzyme levels.
- ◆ Targeting multiple cholesterol issues is a complex issue that requires close monitoring of a patient's health.

Glossary

angiogram   One technique that has been used to identify localized plaque rupture.

angioplasty   Performed to open a narrowed artery. In this procedure, a balloon is opened inside the artery and moves the cholesterol or plaque out of the opening of the blood vessel. A *stent*, something that looks like chicken wire, may be placed in the blood vessel during angioplasty to prevent renarrowing.

antioxidants   Compounds that occur naturally in the body. They help to prevent damage caused by charged compounds called *oxidants*, which are also a natural byproduct of the metabolic process. One type of damaging oxidant is called *free radicals*.

aorta   The main artery that comes off the heart. It supplies blood to the brain, lower extremities, upper extremities, heart, kidneys, and all other organs within the body.

apheresis   A technique by which LDL is physically removed from the blood stream using a machine that separates the LDL and some other adverse cholesterol subfractions from the blood. Apheresis is also called *LDL filtration*.

APO A   The name given to the protein that coats HDL, or the good cholesterol. APO A facilitates the removal of harmful cholesterol in the blood vessels.

arrhythmia   Abnormal heart rhythm. There are several different forms of arrhythmias; some are lethal, and others are relatively harmless. Caffeine-induced arrhythmias, such as premature ventricular contractions (PVCs), are generally benign.

atherosclerosis   A narrowing of the arteries caused by the deposit of cholesterol, dead and dying cells on the blood vessel wall. This narrows the lumen (opening) of the blood vessel. In time, the artery can become completely blocked.

autonomic nervous system   The branch of the nervous that controls involuntary body functions, like the beating of our hearts.

baseline risk   A measurement of risk for heart attack and stroke that is determined by evaluating the risk for developing these conditions, such as diet, exercise, gender, age, and genetics. If a baseline risk is already high, an elevated cholesterol level can make matters even worse.

bile acid sequestrants   A class of medications used to lower cholesterol. *See* resins.

biofeedback   A technique in which a person concentrates on breathing, heartbeat, and blood pressure in an attempt to consciously modify these functions. Biofeedback may allow us to consciously control our autonomic nervous system, which controls involuntary body functions, such as breathing.

calcification   A process wherein calcium salts and compounds are deposited within the cholesterol plaque. This process is thought to actually make the cholesterol plaque more stable and less likely to rupture, but suggests advanced disease.

calorie   A measure of how much potential energy is in a particular food. The definition of a calorie for biological systems is the amount of energy necessary to raise 1,000 grams of water by 1 degree centigrade. Utilizing this definition, all foods can be compared to one another based upon how much energy is stored within the food.

carcinogen   A substance that can cause cancer.

carotenoids   A plant pigments that may help prevent cancer and other conditions related to aging. There are three main types: lycopene, luteins, and beta carotene.

cholesterol   A fatty substance that does not dissolve in the bloodstream. Although cholesterol is needed for some of the body's basic functions, it can also pose serious health risks if it damages the blood vessels.

cholesterol panel   Measures the amount of fatty substances, or lipids, in the blood. The substances measured in a cholesterol panel include HDL, LDL, and triglycerides, and are sometimes referred to as subfractions or lipid subfractions.

coronary CT (computerized tomography)   A technique wherein the amount of calcium within the coronary arteries is quantified.

CRP (C-reactive protein)   A protein made by the liver and reflects the overall level of inflammation in the body. Various stimuli, including infection, may increase CRP, and as the CRP increases, so does your risk for heart attack and stroke.

cytokines   Inflammatory substances released by cells when fighting infection. Cytokines also play a part in the development of atherosclerosis.

DASH (Dietary Approaches to Stop Hypertension)   A healthy diet consisting of fruits and vegetables. The diet was first introduced to reduce high blood pressure, but has also shown promising effects toward lowering cholesterol.

enzyme   A protein that is used to help promote a particular reaction in a cell as part of the cell's metabolism. Elevated enzyme levels may indicate injury or damage in a particular organ.

essential fatty acids   Fatty compounds that are necessary for basic cell functions.

familial hypercholesterolemia   A type of severe cholesterol elevation caused by a genetic defect in the liver. Because LDL can't be removed from the circulation by the liver LDL receptor, it deposits itself elsewhere in the body.

fasting cholesterol panel   A simple blood test obtained after a person has gone 8–12 hours without eating. It eliminates any error associated with raised triglyceride levels caused by eating and gives your doctor a clear idea of which cholesterol sub-fractions may be legitimately elevated.

fasting glucose level   Measures the amount of sugar in the bloodstream and is often obtained along with a fasting cholesterol panel. Elevated glucose levels may mean that a person is diabetic or prediabetic. These conditions pose a threat to cardiovascular health, especially when combined with other risk factors (such as elevated cholesterol levels).

fibric acids   A class of medications used to lower triglycerides and elevate HDL.

fibrin strands   Fibers that enmesh themselves and trap platelets inside of blood clots.

fight or flight   A response that is the body's reaction to feeling threatened. This reaction is powered by the sympathetic nervous system and fueled by adrenaline. In the short term, this is a protective measure, but if you're stressed all the time, it can be harmful to your health.

free radicals   One damaging type of *oxidant*, which are a natural byproduct of metabolism.

French paradox   Refers to a relatively low incidence of heart disease in a population that also consumes a diet rather high in fat and calories.

functional foods   Those foods that help to improve health. These foods may lower cholesterol, lower the incidence of cancer, prevent heart attack, or help to fight blood clots. Some functional foods are believed to have anticarcinogenic, or cancer-fighting effects.

genes   Long DNA molecules that are located on chromosomes. The chromosomes are located in the center of all human cells. There are 23 pairs of human chromosomes in the nucleus (or central command center) of each and every human cell.

gene therapy   Seeks to isolate one defective gene and change it, thus alleviating any illness it has been causing.

heart failure   A term used to describe a condition in which the heart's can't deliver adequate blood, nutrients, and oxygen to the tissues in an effective way.

HDL (high-density lipoprotein)   HDL is believed to play a protective role in the bloodstream, cleaning up the plaque that LDL leaves behind.

heart rate variability study   A study that evaluates the measure of balance between the parasympathetic and sympathetic nervous systems. Normally, the parasympathetic system should be dominant in this balance.

inflammation   The body's response to an infection and other insults. Many different types of cells may be involved in the body's response to inflammation; one type, called macrophages, are sent out to control the bacteria and shut down the infection. Macrophages can also play a role in plaque rupture and subsequent heart attack. Cholesterol can also act as an inflammatory substance and cause inflammation.

insulin resistance   The body's inability to use insulin to convert into other products. The cells of the body become insensitive to insulin, requiring higher insulin levels to maintain a normal blood glue.

intermediates   Substances created during cell metabolism and participant in the harnessing of energy. The energy is transferred in the form of electrons from one intermediate to another.

isoflavones   One type of phytoestrogens. Phytoestrogens are substances found in soy that may have cancer-fighting effects and also help to dilate blood vessels.

isometric exercise   Resistance training, or using a weight or load to condition muscles.

isotonic exercise   Aerobic conditioning, or strengthening the heart and cardiovascular system.

LDL filtration   Also known as *apheresis*, a technique by which LDL is physically removed from the blood stream using a machine that separates the LDL and some other adverse cholesterol subfractions using columns of beads that bind the LDL and other components, such as VLDL.

LDL (low-density lipoprotein)   The role of LDL is to move cholesterol and other fatty compounds that are in excess to places where it can be stored.

lipid   A synonym for fat. When we talk about lipid subfractions, we're talking about the various fatty substances that are floating around in the bloodstream, such as HDL, LDL, and triglycerides. A *cholesterol panel* is a lipid panel—it measures the fat circulating in the blood.

lipoproteins   Combinations of lipids and proteins. All of the cholesterol panel subfractions circulate in the blood as combinations of lipids and proteins.

meditation   A method of gaining control of negative thoughts and training the mind to react in a controlled fashion. The basic principle of meditation is to focus thoughts and concentration on one item to relieve stress.

mental stress test   A test that measures how a person's heart responds to situations of increasing emotional stress and can predict the likelihood of a person developing a heart attack or stroke under similar emotional circumstances.

metabolic syndrome   A group of health issues that raises a person's risk for developing heart attack and stroke. Elevated triglycerides are one element of the metabolic syndrome.

metabolism   The process by which food and other substances, such as medications, are broken down into their most basic components in the body.

moderate alcohol consumption   The consumption of one to two drinks per day for a man and one drink per day for a woman. A drink is defined as a 12-ounce beer, 5 ounces of wine, or 1¼ to 1½ ounces of liquor. Approximately seven drinks per week is considered moderate.

monounsaturated fats   One fewer hydrogen atom than saturated fats have and are somewhat healthier for the heart (at least when used in moderation).

niacin   A B vitamin. When used in low doses, it acts as a vitamin; when used in higher doses, it can help to lower LDL and triglycerides and raise HDL.

non-HDL cholesterol   Any lipoprotein that is not HDL. In addition to LDL and triglycerides, your doctor may be interested in looking at your levels of VLDL (very low-density lipoprotein) and IDL (intermediate-density lipoprotein) levels, both of which increase the risk of heart disease in high levels.

oxidant   A natural byproduct of metabolism. One type of damaging oxidant is called *free radicals*.

oxidized LDL   A particularly dangerous form of LDL. It acts as a magnet, pulling inflammatory cells toward it. The inflammation results in a burst of toxins which damages blood vessel walls.

Paleolithic diet   A diet that basically consists of food that can be found in nature (plants, animals, grains, etc.) It promotes low incidences of diabetes, heart disease, and cancer.

platelet activating factor (PAF)   An inflammatory substance released by platelets which contributes to platelet aggregation, clotting, and other inflammatory responses.

parasympathetic nervous system   A branch of the nervous system that works in balance with the sympathetic nervous system. While the sympathetic nervous system makes the body work harder, the parasympathetic nervous system slows things down and has a more relaxing effect on the body.

physical fitness   A term that describes how much exercise a person can tolerate.

phytoestrogens   Protective compounds found in soy that promote dilation of blood vessels and protect against heart disease and certain cancers. *Isoflavones* are one type of phytoestrogens.

placebo effect   The belief that a certain therapy has worked because a person thought that it would, despite evidence suggesting that the therapy may not work.

plaque   Forms on blood vessel walls. It's made up of a liquid pool containing cholesterol and by-products of inflammation as well as a protective cap that prevents the cholesterol from entering into the blood stream.

plaque volume   The amount of space the plaque occupies in three-dimensional space.

platelets   Small disc-like cells in the bloodstream. Platelets are smaller than other blood cells and float through the blood searching for an injured area. These cells release an inflammatory compound called *platelet activating factor*, or *PAF*, which contributes to the formation of blood clots.

pleiotropic   Benefits that certain medications may provide over and above what they're primarily used for. Statins are thought to have pleiotropic effects: They raise HDL, lower LDL, and help stimulate progenitor cells, a type of cell that helps to rebuild damaged heart cells.

prostaglandins   Substances that either dilate (open) or constrict (close) blood vessels. Omega-3 fatty acids in the membranes of platelets create a situation in which there are more dilatory prostaglandins present.

resins   A class of medications that interfere with the cycling of cholesterol from the liver to the digestive tract and back. These are also called bile acid resins or *bile acid sequestrants.*

restenosis   Refers to the renarrowing of an artery that has already been opened by *angioplasty.*

risk/benefit ratio   Refers to your doctor weighing the benefits of a particular course of treatment against the possibility of a negative outcome.

risk factor   A behavior, lifestyle, or other factor that increases a person's likelihood of developing a disease or condition.

risk factor modification   Involves evaluating your various risk factors and changing them as needed to lower your chances of developing illness.

risk factor score   A numerical assessment of a person's multiple risk factors for heart disease and stroke. One major consideration in this score is a person's cholesterol levels. The final score indicates the probability of developing heart disease or stroke in the future.

statins   One class of medications that doctors use to treat cholesterol disorders. These are very safe drugs whose primary mechanism of action is to remove LDL from the bloodstream.

stenosis   A narrowing of an artery. (Several narrowings are called *stenoses.*) The blood vessels will sometimes compensate for a stenosis by developing collaterals around the blockage or by actually increasing in diameter.

stent Something that looks like chicken wire, may be placed in the blood vessel during angioplasty to prevent renarrowing.

sympathetic nervous system A branch of the nervous system that makes organs work harder and fuels the fight-or-flight response a person has when he or she feels threatened. The *parasympathetic nervous system* has a more relaxing effect on the body.

triglycerides Fatty substances that circulate in the bloodstream. Although triglycerides are routinely measured in a *cholesterol panel*, their chemical makeup and basic functions differ from cholesterol.

vascular endothelial growth factor (VEGF) A compound responsible for the sprouting of new blood vessels. It's also responsible for allowing some cancers to metastasize. Researchers are currently looking for a way to harness VEGF's properties to allow new blood vessel growth around the scar tissue left by a heart attack.

Appendix B

Further Reading

American Heart Association, et al. *American Heart Association Low-Fat, Low-Cholesterol Cookbook, 3rd ed.* New York: Crown Publishing Group, 2004.

Appel, L. J., et al. "A clinical trial of the effects of dietary patterns on blood pressure. DASH Collaborative Research Group." *New England Journal of Medicine* 336 (1997): 1117-24.

Assouline, L., et al. "Familial hypercholesterolemia: molecular, biochemical, and clinical characterization of a French-Canadian pediatric population." *Pediatrics* 96 (2 Pt 1): 239-46 (1995).

Baum, Seth J., M.D. *The Total Guide to a Healthy Heart, Integrative Strategies for Preventing and Reversing Heart Disease.* New York: Kensington Publishing Corp., 1999.

Cannon, Christopher, M.D., ed. *Management of Acute Coronary Syndromes.* Totowa, NJ: Humana Press, 1999.

Cobb, M. M., H. S. Teitelbaum, and J. L. Breslow. "Lovastatin efficacy in reducing low-density lipoprotein cholesterol levels on high- vs. low-fat diets." *JAMA* 265 (1991): 997-1001.

Cooke, John P., M.D. *The Cardiovascular Cure, How to Strengthen Your Self Defense Against Heart Attack and Stroke.* New York: Broadway Books, 2002.

Cordain, Loren. *The Paleo Diet.* Hoboken: John Wiley & Sons Inc., 2002.

Criqui, M.H., and B. L. Ringel. "Does diet or alcohol explain the French paradox?" *Lancet* 344 (1994): 1719-23.

Davich, Victor N. *8 Minute Meditation: Quiet Your Mind. Change Your Life.* New York: Berkley, 2004.

de Lorgeril, M., et al. "Mediterranean alpha-linoleic acid rich diet in secondary prevention of coronary heart disease." *Lancet* 343 (1994): 1454-59.

Denke, M. A. "Cholesterol-Lowering diets: review of the evidence." *Archives of Internal Medicine* 155 (1995): 17-26.

———. "Review of human studies evaluating individual dietary responsiveness in patient with hypercholesterolemia." *American Journal of Clinical Nutrition* 62 (1995): 471S-477S.

Denke, M. A.; and S. M. Grundy. "Individual responses to a cholesterol-lowering diet in 50 men with moderate hypercholesterolemia." *Archives of Internal Medicine* 154 (1994): 317-25.

Denke, M. A., C. T. Sempos, and S. M. Grundy. "Excess body weight: an under-recognized contributor to dyslipidemia in white American women." *Archives of Internal Medicine* 154 (1994): 401-10.

———. "Excess body weight: an under-recognized contributor to high blood cholesterol levels in white American men.: *Archives of Internal Medicine* 154 (1993): 1093-1103.

GISSI-Prevenzione Investigators. "Dietary supplementation with n-3 polyunsaturated fatty acids and vitamin E after myocardial infarction: results of the GISSI-Prevenzione trial." *Lancet* 354 (1999): 447-55.

Grundy, S. M. "Small LDL, atherogenic dyslipidemia, and the metabolic syndrome." *Circulation* 95 (1997): 1-4.

Hegsted, D. M., et al. "Quantitative effects of dietary fat on serum cholesterol levels in man." *American Journal of Clinical Nutrition* 17 (1995): 281-95.

Hjermann, I, I. Holme, and P. Leren. "Oslo Study Diet and Anti-Smoking Trial: results after 102 months." *American Journal of Medicine* 80 [Suppl 2A]: 7-12 (1986).

Hunninghake, D. B., et al. "The efficacy of intensive dietary therapy alone or combined with lovastatin in outpatients with hypercholesterolemia." *New England Journal of Medicine* 328 (1993): 1213-19.

Kato, H., et al. "Epidemiologic studies of coronary heart disease and stroke in Japanese men living in Japan, Hawaii and California." *American Journal of Epidemiology* 97 (1973): 372-85.

Law, M., and N. Wald. "Why heart disease mortality is low in France: the time lag explanation." *BMJ* 318 (1999): 1471-80.

Lichtenstein, A. H., et al. "Hydrogenation impairs the hypolipidemic effect of corn oil in humans: hydrogenation, trans fatty acids, and plasma lipids." *Arteriosclerosis and Thrombosis* 13 (1993): 154-61.

Multiple Risk Factor Intervention Trial Research Group. "Multiple Risk factor Intervention Trial; risk factor changes and mortality results." *JAMA* 248 (1982): 1465-77.

National Cholesterol Education Program. Adult Treatment Panel III, May 2001.

Ornish, D., et al. "Can lifestyle changes reverse coronary heart disease? The Lifestyle Heart Trial." *Lancet* 335 (1990): 129-33.

Reaven, Gerald, M.D. *Syndrome X, Overcoming the Silent Killer That Can Give You a Heart Attack*. New York: Simon & Schuster, 2000.

Robertson, T. I., et al. "Epidemiology studies of coronary heart disease and stroke in Japanese men living in Japan, Hawaii, and California." *American Journal of Cardiology* 39 (1997): 239-43.

Schuler, G., et al. "Regular physical exercise and low-fat diet: effects of progression on coronary artery disease." *Circulation* 86 (1992): 1-11.

Schlosser, Eric. *Fast Food Nation: The Dark Side of the All-American Meal*. New York: Houghton Mifflin, 2001.

Shekelle, R.B., et al. "Diet, serum cholesterol, and death from coronary heart disease: the Western Electric Study." *New England Journal of Medicine* 304 (1981): 65-70.

Stamler, J., and R. Shekell. "Dietary cholesterol and human coronary heart disease." *Archives of Pathology and Laboratory Medicine* 112 (1988): 1032-40.

Swenson, David A. *Ashtanga Yoga: The Practice Manual: An Illustrated Guide to Personal Practice*. Austin: Ashtanga Yoga Productions, 1999.

Turpeinem, O., et al. "Dietary prevention of heart disease: The Finish Mental Hospital Study." *International Journal of Epidemiology* 8 (1979): 99-118.

Watts, G. F., et al. "Effects of coronary artery disease of lipid lowering diet, or diet plus cholestyramine in the St. Thomas Atherosclerosis Regression Study (STARS)." *Lancet* 339 (1992): 563-69.

Wilhelmsen, L., et al. "The Multi-factor Primary Prevention Trial in Goteborg, Sweden." *European Heart Journal* 7 (1986): 277-88.

World Health Organization Collaborative Group. "Multifactorial trial in the prevention of coronary heart disease III. Incidence and mortality results." *European Heart Journal* 4 (1983): 141-47.

Heart-Healthy Recipes

Because the recipes listed in this appendix are easy to prepare (honest!), they're perfect for those of you who'd rather *not* be stuck in the kitchen for hours on end. They're also a great way to introduce yourself to the flavor-boosters that are commonly used in low-fat cooking, like herbs, spices, and low-fat ingredients like vinegar and mustard. Feel free to experiment with different low-fat accoutrements in these recipes (a different type of herb might be more to your liking, for example). Remember, variety is the spice of life, and it can add a real kick to your cooking, too!

Main Dishes

Grilled Fish with Vegetables

Serves 4
Prep time: about an hour
Cook time: 10 minutes
Total time: 1 hour, 15 minutes
Serving size: 1 fillet

2 large mushrooms

1 medium bell pepper

1 small onion

2 TB. marjoram or basil

3 TB. water

3 TB. balsamic or cider vinegar

1 TB. olive oil

¼ tsp. pepper

4 (6-oz.) fillets white fish (like snapper, dogfish, or halibut)

Nonstick cooking spray

1. Wash vegetables. Using a sharp knife, slice mushrooms into thin pieces. Cut pepper in half lengthwise; remove membrane and seeds; cut into thin strips. Slice onion into thin strips.

2. Whisk marjoram or basil with water, vinegar, olive oil, and pepper. Add veggies to the mix and refrigerate for one hour.

3. Preheat the grill.

4. Create a foil packet for veggies: take a strip of foil measuring about 18 inches wide by 12 inches long. Fold in half lengthwise; fold the shorter outside edges over twice.

5. Remove veggies from marinade, taking care to reserve some marinade for the fish. Place veggies into remaining opening of the foil packet. Fold the last opening over twice to close the packet.

6. When ready to grill, spray grill with nonstick cooking spray. Using a metal spatula, place foil packet on grill for 8–10 minutes.

7. Use remaining marinade to coat both sides of each fish fillet. Grill about 5 minutes on each side or until fish flakes easily with a fork.

8. Remove veggie packet with metal spatula. Serve as a side dish or spoon on top of each fillet.

Baked Lemony Trout

3 lemons

¼ cup minced basil, dill, or tarragon

2 tsp. olive oil

4 (4-oz.) rainbow-trout fillets

Nonstick cooking spray

Pepper to taste

Serves 4
Prep time: 15 minutes
Cook time: 15 minutes
Total time: 30 minutes
Serving size: 1 fillet

1. Preheat oven to 350°F.

2. Slice one lemon into ¼-inch rings. Cut the other two lemons in half. Over a small bowl, squeeze juice from the four halves.

3. Combine herbs and olive oil in the bowl with lemon juice. Set aside.

4. Cover sides and bottom of a 9×13-inch casserole dish with tin-foil; spray with nonstick cooking spray. Place lemon slices on the bottom of the casserole dish; lay fillets over lemon slices.

5. Pour lemon juice/herb/olive oil mixture over fillets.

6. Bake for 12–15 minutes or until fish flakes easily with a fork.

Summer Squash Stir-Fry

6 cups cooked brown rice

½ cup low-sodium chicken broth

½ tsp. crushed garlic

2 medium zucchini, sliced

2 medium yellow squash, sliced

1 medium onion, chopped

1 large tomato, peeled and chopped

1–2 TB. balsamic vinegar

½ tsp. pepper

6 cups cooked brown rice

Serves 5
Prep time: 15 minutes
Cook time: 15 minutes
Total time: 30 minutes
Serving size: ½ cup

1. Preheat large skillet over medium heat for 1 minute. Add broth and garlic and stir for about 1 minute.

2. Add the zucchini, yellow squash, and onion. Stir-fry for 3–4 minutes.

3. Add tomato, vinegar, and pepper. Reduce to a simmer. Stir occasionally until vegetables are tender. Serve over brown rice.

Lentil Soup

Serves 8
Prep time: 30 minutes
Cook time: 1 hour
Total time: 1 hour, 30 minutes
Serving size: 1 cup

1 TB. olive oil

1 large onion, diced

2 TB. minced or crushed garlic

2 tsp. curry powder

1½–2 cups chopped tomatoes (may substitute low-salt crushed tomatoes, drained)

2–3 medium carrots, diced

1 stalk celery, sliced

6 cups water

2 cups dried lentils

1. Pour olive oil into a large saucepan; heat over medium-high burner. Add onion and garlic; sauté 2 minutes, until onion starts to soften.

2. Add curry powder and fresh tomatoes, stirring continuously for 3–4 minutes. (If using canned tomatoes, reduce time to 1 minute.)

3. Add water, carrots, celery and lentils. Bring to boil.

4. When mixture is boiling, *partially* cover, making sure to vent the pot. Reduce heat to medium-low. Simmer 1 hour, or until lentils are soft. Serve with whole grain rolls.

Turkey Burgers

Serves 4
Prep time: 10 minutes
Cook time: 10–12 minutes
Total time: about 25 minutes
Serving size: 1 burger

1 lb. ground turkey

1 tsp. dried tarragon

1 TB. finely chopped onion

Nonstick cooking spray

4 whole-wheat sandwich buns

1. Preheat the grill.

2. Combine ground turkey, tarragon, and onion in a medium bowl and mix well.

3. Shape mixture into 4 patties.

4. Spray grill rack with nonstick cooking spray and place patties on grill. Cook over medium heat 10–12 minutes, turning once, or until no pink remains. Serve on whole-wheat buns.

Chicken Fajitas

1 lb. boneless skinless
chicken breast

½ cup balsamic vinegar

1 cup green bell pepper

1 cup red bell pepper

½ cup chopped onion

½ cup grated low-fat cheese

½ cup low-fat plain yogurt

4 soft tortilla shells

2 cups cooked brown rice

Serves 4
Prep time: 10 minutes
Cook time: 20 minutes
Total time: 30 minutes
Serving size: 1 fajita

1. Cut chicken into cubes or strips and marinate in vinegar.

2. Cut peppers and onion into strips.

3. Spray a large skillet with nonstick vegetable spray. Add peppers and onions, and sauté for 8–10 minutes until soft.

4. Add chicken and cook uncovered, stirring occasionally until no pink remains.

5. Divide chicken-and-vegetable mixture among tortilla shells. Add a sprinkle of low-fat cheese if desired, and a dollop of plain low fat yogurt. Serve with ½ cup of brown rice on the side.

Orange Beef and Vegetables

2 medium seedless oranges

4 cups cooked brown rice

1 TB. olive oil

1 (12 oz.) lean top round
steak, thinly sliced

1 (10 oz.) bag frozen veggies

Serves 4
Prep time: 10 minutes
Cook time: about 12–15 minutes
Total time: 25–30 minutes
Serving size: 1 cup

1. Grate peel of one orange and set aside. Cut both oranges in half. Over a small bowl, squeeze juice from the four halves and set aside.

2. Heat olive oil in a skillet over medium heat. Add beef and stir-fry until no longer pink, about 5–6 minutes. Remove beef from the skillet and set aside.

3. Add frozen veggies, orange juice, and orange peel to the skillet. Cook for 4 minutes, stirring continuously.

4. Add beef back into mixture in the skillet; stir-fry for 1 minute or until beef is reheated. Serve over brown rice.

Side Dishes

Mango-Pineapple Salsa

Serves 3
Prep time: 20 minutes, plus 1–4 hours refrigeration time
Cook time: none
Serving size: 1 cup

1 cup pineapple chunks

¾ cup peeled pitted mango, diced

⅔ cup diced red bell pepper

½ cup diced seeded tomato

⅓ cup seeded English hothouse cucumber

⅓ cup diced red onion

3 TB. minced fresh cilantro (optional)

2 TB. minced fresh mint (optional)

2 TB. fresh lime juice

1. Combine ingredients in medium bowl. Chill to blend flavors, at least 1 hour and up to 4 hours, tossing occasionally.

2. Serve over grilled fish or as a dip with melba toast.

Healthy Coleslaw

Serves 4
Prep time: 15 minutes plus 2–3 hours to chill
Cook time: none
Serving size: 1 cup

1 (32-oz.) package preshredded coleslaw mix

1 cup plain low-fat yogurt

¼ cup low-fat buttermilk

1 TB. cider vinegar

1 tsp. Dijon mustard

1 pinch cayenne pepper

Black pepper to taste

1 shredded carrot (garnish, optional)

1. Combine low-fat yogurt, low-fat buttermilk, cider vinegar, Dijon mustard, cayenne pepper, and black pepper and whisk until smooth, or prepare in a food processor or blender.

2. Toss cabbage mix with dressing and allow to marinate for 2–3 hours or overnight.

3. Serve chilled, garnished with shredded carrot (if desired).

Desserts/Snacks

Fruit Smoothie

½ **cup skim milk**

½ **cup nonfat yogurt**

½ **cup orange juice**

½ **frozen banana, peeled**

½ **cup frozen strawberries**

Serves 1
Prep time: 5 minutes
Cook time: none
Serving size: 1 cup

1. Combine all ingredients in a blender; blend on high until smooth.

Baked Apples

4 apples (not a tart variety)

2 cups water

½ **cup honey**

½ **cup raisins or currants**

½ **cup walnuts**

1 tsp. cinnamon or nutmeg

Serves 4
Prep time: 15 minutes
Cook time: 1 hour
Serving size: 1 apple

1. Preheat oven to 350°F.

2. Pour water into the bottom of a pie dish.

3. Core the apples, leaving the bottom intact. (A melon-baller is a useful tool here.)

4. Mix honey, raisins or currants, walnuts, and cinnamon or nutmeg together in a small bowl. Spoon mixture into each apple.

5. Bake for about an hour, until apples are softened. (Cooking time may vary depending on the size of the apples; when the apples start to smell like they're done, you'll know they're getting close!)

Fruit and Yogurt Parfait

Serves 1
Prep time: 10 minutes
Cook time: none
Serving size: 1 parfait

1 cup vanilla low-fat yogurt
¼ cup strawberries
¼ cup blueberries

¼ cup chopped peaches
¼ cup crushed, drained pineapple

1. Spread ¼ cup yogurt in the bottom of a 10-ounce glass.
2. Layer strawberries on top of yogurt.
3. Layer another ¼ cup yogurt on top of the strawberries.
4. Follow with blueberries.
5. Layer ¼ cup yogurt on top of blueberries.
6. Follow with peaches.
7. Layer ¼ cup yogurt on top of peaches.
8. Top off with crushed pineapple.

Index

E

G

I

oxidants, 103, 119, 216
    antioxidants, 219-220
    damage process, 216-217
        periods of vulnerability, 219
        plaque, 217-218
        plaque volume increase, 218-219
oxidized LDLs, 21

P–Q

PAF (platelet-activating factor), capsicum, 197
Paleolithic diets, 52, 77
    developing lifelong programs, 124
    lifestyle changes, 78
    modern changes, 78-79
    sample menus, 81-82
palm kernel oils, 76
palm oils, 76
palmitic acids, 39
pantetheine, 208-209
parasympathetic nervous systems
    adrenaline system, 154
    balance with sympathetic nervous system, 165-166
parents, healthy influence on children, 235
peanuts, HDL booster, 33
pecans, HDL booster, 33
phenolic acids, 92
physical activities. *See also* exercise
    assessing current condition, 134
    changeable risk factors, 53-54
    cholesterol effects, 134-135
    deloping lifelong healthy eating, 125
    encouraging for children, 235-236
    healthy living guide, 236-237
        aerobic with resistance exercise, 238
        daily routine, 237-238
    heart
        condition, 136
        failure classifications, 136-137
    measuring current level, 135-136
    medical physicals, 137-138
    prescriptions, 141-142

program building, 142
    basics of weight training, 148-149
    healthy living guide, medical exam, 238-239
    isometric exercises, 142
    isotonic exercises, 143
    levels, 143-146
    medical examination, 149
    resistance training, 146-148
risk factors, 12
slow change in activity level, 135
staging heart failure, 137
stimulating HDLs, 33
two-pronged approach, 138-139
    benefits, 138-139
    positive effects, 139-140
physical fitness
    assessing current condition, 134
    cholesterol effects, 134-135
    heart condition, 136
    heart failure classifications, 136-137
    measuring current level, 135-136
    medical physicals, 137-138
    slow change in activity level, 135
    staging heart failure, 137
    two-pronged approach, 138-140
physicals, pre-exercise checkups, 137-138
phytic acids, 92
phytochemicals
    functional foods, 92
    green tea, 119-120
phytoestrogens, 84
phytosterols, 92
placebo effects, mind, 154-155
plaque, 9
    oxidants, 217-218
    reduction with statins, 175
    size reduction developments, 225
    stabilizing, 220
    volume, 218-219, 224
platelet-activating factor (PAF), capsicum, 197
platelets, 197
pleiotropic effects, statins, 174-175

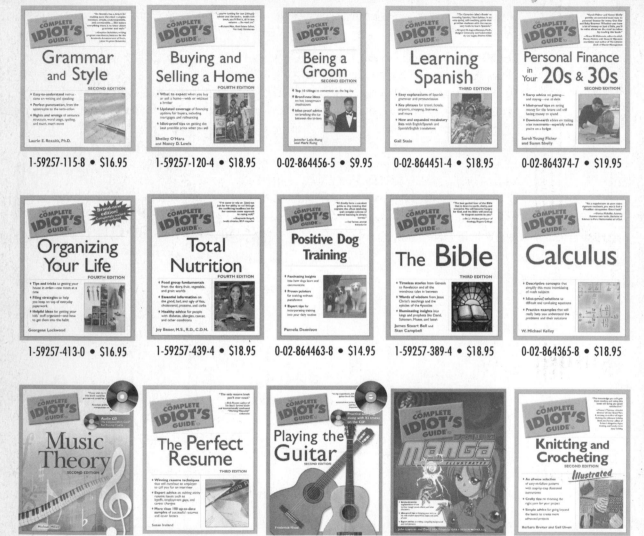